Women, Body, Illness

Women, Body, Illness

Space and Identity in the Everyday Lives of Women with Chronic Illness

Pamela Moss
and
Isabel Dyck

ROWMAN & LITTLEFIELD PUBLISHERS, INC.
Lanham • Boulder • New York • Oxford

ROWMAN & LITTLEFIELD PUBLISHERS, INC.

Published in the United States of America
by Rowman & Littlefield Publishers, Inc.
A Member of the Rowman & Littlefield Publishing Group
4501 Forbes Boulevard, Suite 200, Lanham, Maryland 20706
www.rowmanlittlefield.com

P.O. Box 317, Oxford, OX2 9RU, United Kingdom

British Library Cataloguing in Publication Information Available

The hardback edition of this book was previously cataloged by the Library of Congress as
follows:

Library of Congress Cataloging-in-Publication Data

Moss, Pamela, 1960–
    Women, body, illness : space and identity in the everyday lives of
women with chronic illness / Pamela Moss and Isabel Dyck.
        p. cm.
    Includes bibliographical references and index.
    ISBN 0-8476-9543-3 (alk. paper)
    ISBN 0-8476-9544-1 (pbk. : alk. paper)
    1. Chronic diseases—Psychological aspects.   2. Chronic
diseases—Social aspects.   3. Women—Diseases—Psychological aspects.
4. Women—Diseases—Social aspects.   5. Body image.   6. Spatial
behavior.   7. Social medicine.   8. Feminist theory.   9. Human
geography.   I. Dyck, Isabel.   II. Title.
RC108 .M674   2002
616'.044'082—dc21   2002001197

Printed in the United States of America

♾ ™ The paper used in this publication meets the minimum requirements of American
National Standard for Information Sciences—Permanence of Paper for Printed Library
Materials, ANSI/NISO Z39.48-1992.

*For the women in our lives
who have chronic illness*

Contents

Acknowledgments

This book would not have been possible if it were not for the women talking with us. We wish we could thank you each individually for being part of the project without compromising confidentiality. But we cannot. We know that the time and energy you put into the interviews was physically and emotionally draining. Your stories have assisted us in making sense of chronic illness. We wish you well. You know who you are!

There are several people who have been part of the research for this project: Kathleen Gabelmann, Ann Vanderbilj, Jason Petrunia, Wanda Ollis, Amy Zidulka, and Liisa Peramaki. We thank you for your incredible work skills. Some research from this project has already been presented at conferences and published in academic journals. The feedback we got from audience members and reviewers was useful in sorting through both our ideas about women, bodies, and chronic illness and the women's accounts of their everyday lives. We thank Ken Josephson for translating our thoughts into the visual representations in chapter 4. The Social Science and Humanities Research Council of Canada (SSHRCC) funded this project (No. 410-95-0267).

We also thank everyone at Rowman & Littlefield. We appreciated the patience and professionalism they always showed. Thanks especially to Brenda Hadenfeldt who permitted us time to pull our ideas together in the face of our own everyday lives.

Isabel thanks all those colleagues, students, and friends who in different ways have contributed to her thinking about bodies and chronic illness. In particular, I would like to acknowledge many insightful conversations with Beverley Gartrell. Although they do not appear directly in this book, I would also like to acknowledge the contributions of women with MS from a previous study, whose accounts of their lives with chronic illness have been a continuing personal inspiration as well as setting in motion my participation in this project. My family's ongoing interest in and support for all my endeavors, including this, is something I will always be appreciative of. Thanks go particularly to Sarah and Zoë.

Pamela would like to thank the women (and the few men) who were part of a previous study about seniors living with arthritis. The insight gained into daily life provided the basis for the work included here. I also thank the Geography Department at the University of Vienna, Austria, for support during research leave in the academic year 1998–1999. Thanks to the Faculty of Human and Social Development for support since fall 1999, especially Dean Anita Molzahn, who facilitated a smooth transition to a professional faculty. Students, both inside and outside the classroom, also contributed in the development of my ideas, especially those in the seminars *Spatial and Sexual Politics* in spring 1997, *Women in the City* in spring 1998, and *Women in the Human Services* in spring 2001, all at the University of Victoria. Interaction with graduate students and senior undergraduates over the years around issues of body and chronic illness has been invaluable in writing this book. Thanks to Kathleen, Wanda, Jason, Amy, Andrea Lloyd, Jessica Dempsey, Robin Roth, and Sally Kimpson. My colleagues have also contributed to the writing of the book indirectly through various conversations over the years: Margo Matwychuk, Martha McMahon, Kathy Teghtsoonian, Margot Young, Radhika Desai, David Butz, and Lawrence Berg. Members and Directors of the ME Victoria Association, 1999–2001, showed me ways to live with chronic illness and inspired me to continue working on the project. I especially thank Zosia Lacz, Ken Beattie, Catherine Miller, Rosemary Joy, Simon Perrott, Sid Tukeman, Margaret Sherwood, and Monica Kwas. Thanks, too, to Mae Postnikoff and Phyllis Griffiths for keeping me posted on developments in the field of diagnosing, treating, and living with ME.

Pamela thanks her friends and family. They have supported me and my efforts throughout this project in many ways—from helping with references to reading paragraphs, from giving me rides to providing space to write, from playing Mah-Jongg on Sundays to making me tea almost daily. I could never thank any of you enough—Karl, Ann, Clarice, Hannah, Kath, Kathy, Sam, John, Herbert, Tim, Joan, Elizabeth, Mary, Jason, and Ken.

Prologue

Living with Chronic Illness

Today. What's today? . . . Okay, Wednesday. Two classes, one meeting, no parents, one principal, 20 kids. I wish this body would quit aching. Quick. Take inventory. Ankles, pain. Knees, lots of pain. Hips, okay. Ooh. Thighs, new type of pain. I've got to remember that. Back . . . lower pain, middle okay, upper stiff, neck, only on the left side. Okay. Shoulders, left hurts worse. No blackboard work today. Elbows, stiff. Wrists, fine. Fingers, too stiff to tell. Check later. Danielle works today so I have time to nap this afternoon. . . . Now if I open my eyes . . . everything looks okay. What time is it? Ooh, just fifteen minutes. The light's too bright. I need darker blinds. . . . I'm never going to make it. Point, stretch, flex, hold. Point, stretch, flex, hold. If I get these done, I'll be able to get out of bed easier. Wednesday . . . hum . . . doctor. When is it? 1:15, just after school. Or was it 2:30? The tests should have come back. I wonder. There's got to be something. . . . Music. Danielle's up. Good, I'll at least have some breakfast . . . flex, hold. I can do this. Did I put the garbage out? It's probably too late anyway. . . . Who knows? Maybe she'll believe me this time. It just can't all be in my head. That just doesn't make any sense. Roll over. Up, two, three, four. Up, two, . . . hum . . . I hurt. All over. It's not possible for someone to hurt all over and be tired . . . all the time. For so long. Is it? It can't be. Laundry. Maybe I can get by with just towels today. How long has it been for sheets? If we didn't have to go to Ladysmith tomorrow, there would be plenty of time. No, not tomorrow. Friday. . . . What's today? Wednesday. That's it . . . up, two, three, four . . . Danielle should probably see her grandparents. Ross could take her. Okay fine. Ouch. My hands hurt. That's never happened before. When is this all going to go away? "Yeah, yeah. I'm up. I'll be there in a minute."

Here we introduce Patience, a composite fictional character who exemplifies the life of a woman with chronic illness. We visit Patience throughout the book to illustrate the problems (and triumphs) of the day-to-day existence of women with chronic illness.

Patience has been struggling with illness for almost four years. Within a month, early one fall, her father died, her sister was seriously injured in a car accident, and her husband had told her that he had fallen out of love with her. When she first started feeling weak, after a bout with the flu, she thought it was physical manifestations of stress. And so did her family doctor. Increasingly, she was sluggish and tired throughout the day. She complained of forgetfulness, fatigue, pain. Going to sleep wasn't a problem, staying asleep was. The doctor suggested that she was depressed, and prescribed anti-depressants. Given how close she had been to her family and how devastated she was knowing that her husband didn't love her anymore, depression made sense. She also knew that once stress started "coming out," it could take a long time to get over.

Months passed. Patience wasn't quite sure what to do about the marriage, so she carried on as if nothing had changed. She had married straight out of high school to a man several years older. Their leisure revolved around outdoor activities. They bought a house and moved to the suburbs to live among friends with whom they could ski, camp, hike, kayak, and cycle. While her husband built his career, she decided to go to university to become an elementary school teacher. She earned a B.A. in sociology, graduating with honors. Just before she completed the teaching certificate program, she had a child, Danielle. Soon thereafter, Patience landed a job with the local school board and taught full-time. Her marriage was traditional in the sense that she took care of everything in the household, from cleaning to childcare, from shopping to emotional support, from planning holidays to taking out the garbage. For years she lived a life that she thought she had always wanted—family, house, friends, career.

Then her father died unexpectedly from a stroke when she was 36. Because she had always been closer to her mother, the death of her father hit her harder emotionally than she had expected. Just when she thought that she had adjusted to the fact he was dead, her sister was injured in a head-on collision. For two weeks, Jenny lay in hospital recovering from both the multiple leg and hip fractures and the surgeries needed to reduce the visible effects of scarring to the face and arms. Emotional ties to the women closest to her obliged Patience to work through the grief that accompanies the death of a spouse of forty-four years with her mother and the angst that surfaces when trying to come to terms with visible disfigurement and altered mobility with her sister. Responsibility of comforting rested on Patience for she was furthest removed from the immediacy of distress. However, exactly one month after her father's death, her husband told her he no longer loved her and felt that she should know.

Just one more set of stretches. Sit up. Left side. Stretch. . . . And five more minutes. Ooh, got to hurry. . . . I know I could be better if I didn't have to stay in touch with him. Such bad timing for a break up. . . . A break up. I would've never thought. . . . And that woman . . . I wonder if she knows him very well. I know I'm better off without him. She probably would be too. It would've been impossible to change with him around. . . . Do I want to change? . . . Change. . . . Of course I do. If only my body would stop falling apart. . . . It would have been more and more pressure. . . . Maybe there's someone else who I could be with. He found someone else, why can't I? . . . If Danielle had only been older. How am I going to do it? . . . Switch sides. Ouch, that's sore. I wonder if it's only aging? . . . How does anyone ever endure getting older? . . . How does anyone ever find someone to be with if you have a body like mine?

Instead of collapsing, Patience persevered. She continued to teach full-time, care for Danielle who was 11 at the time, maintain the household, provide support for her mother and sister, and live in a relationship in limbo. At the onset of her symptoms, concurrent with the series of emotional upsets, she chose not to tell anyone. There seemed too much going on without further complicating matters with a nebulous illness. Rather than engaging in after-school activities, she feigned family commitments and went home to rest. Because cycling jolted her bones and kayaking frayed her muscles, she began distancing herself from her active friends. Initially, the extra social space appeared to be a result of the death and the accident. However, her friends became frustrated with Patience for canceling outings at the last minute or being too busy even to meet. She began phoning her mother rather than dropping by; and she saw her sister less frequently, relying on e-mail. After a year or so, she began withdrawing even further from her family, telling them she was busy at school. She stayed in contact with a small circle of friends, ones whom she did not relate to through outdoor activities. She simply ignored the emotional distance between herself and her husband and pretended that everything was, and would be, fine.

Two years after the onset of symptoms and the deluge of emotional stress, Patience decided that she could not work full-time anymore. Instead of utilizing the sick leave or long-term disability policy, she negotiated a .4 FTE (full-time equivalency), which included three class periods daily. In addition to teaching in the classroom, these class periods included time for course preparation and meetings. She reasoned that the reduction in hours, arranged so that she could regenerate herself on a daily basis from the primary symptoms of pain and fatigue, would make up for the reduced income because she could count, at least for now, on the financial stability of her husband's career. This extra time, too, might give her time to re-establish a relationship with her husband. A few months after settling her work arrangements, her husband told her he had fallen in love with another woman, wanted a divorce, and moved out. As part of the divorce settlement, he sued for full custody of Danielle and half the money from the sale of the house.

For just over a year, Patience contested the proposed settlement. She countersued for all the money from the sale of the house, full custody, and support payments for herself and Danielle. They eventually settled by splitting all assets and sharing joint custody, with Patience handling support payments from Ross for Danielle.

I've got to keep telling myself that that this move has been good. For Danielle. For me. And I don't have to worry about Ross anymore. Good. What could be better? . . . Right side. . . . Wow, this is a lot easier. . . . I don't think I put out the garbage. Danielle . . . she used to be so sweet. . . . She's really smart. . . . Is that working? This is the last set, why can't I get it? . . . I remember fighting with my mom, too. But I don't remember it being so nasty. I don't remember being so sassy. . . . Sassy. . . . Maybe I should bring Danielle with me to the doctor. Maybe she would have some, well, interesting things to say to the doctor. . . . Would that be a treat! . . . One last stretch. . . . All right . . . I'm up. . . . What? It's Tuesday? . . . It's Tuesday. Damn.

Patience moved from the split-level into a three-bedroom rancher. Even though she would have liked to have stayed near the old house to be close to some friends, Patience thought that by changing neighborhoods, she could cut some unappealing ties with her now ex-husband. Danielle's not wanting to change schools limited the range of possible moves, and restricted Patience's choice in whether to rent or own. In the end, she rented at a little above market price so that Danielle could walk to school and so that she would have a short drive to work. Because of the change in residence, Patience had to cut back even more of her social contacts, including her book club from university days which met every other month. Family members were no longer routinely part of her life. She narrowly focused what energy she had on Danielle and the specific set of tasks that would get her through a half-day of teaching four days a week.

At the end of the last school year, six months ago, Patience and Danielle began a new phase in their mother-daughter relationship. Because Danielle had chosen to live with her mother during the week, she and Patience had to work out a new system to live together by sharing responsibilities around the house. Patience no longer had the income to hire biweekly housekeepers so she and Danielle became more like roommates negotiating cleaning schedules for common areas. Danielle took on the heavier work that could be done every two or three weeks, like vacuuming, cleaning the bathroom and kitchen, and hand-wash laundry. Patience was responsible for cooking dinner, grocery shopping, meal preparation, regular laundry, and putting out the garbage and recyclables. Though not ideal for either one, this arrangement worked until school began in the fall. Mornings became more difficult for Patience and she asked if Danielle would take on making breakfast in the morning. The trade-off was that Patience would drive Danielle to work and pick her up at the end of her shift. This shift caused more tension between them, especially with regard to resentment over time commitments for both of them—Patience spent more time driving and Danielle had to get up earlier.

Let me think . . . Zoloft . . . I wonder where that name came from? Zo . . . Zo . . . Zoë. I wonder how's she doing. I should call her. . . . No. I just can't. She talks so much and I can never get away. But I really should phone. Maybe next week. "Yes! I'll be out in a minute." *Of what little time I spend in the bathroom. . . .* "I thought you were already in here!" *Is this the most important place in the world? I'm glad I'm not 14. No, it's 15. She's 15! Oh my. And I'm 40. . . . Dark circles. I don't ever remember thinking about being 40. And I certainly never thought I'd feel this way. Not until I was older at least. What an effort to wear make-up. . . . Nope, no curling iron today. . . . I wonder if I can do it with my other hand. . . . This stupid shoulder. . . . I think straight hair is just fine. Quite attractive. . . . Wednesday! Danielle's not working. She usually works, but not this week. Or is it tomorrow? I'd better ask. I hate this getting up. It's too quick. It's going to be a long day. . . . I'm never going to make it.*

Throughout this time, Patience regularly consulted her family doctor. In addition to the anti-depressants, her doctor had prescribed anti-anxiety medication and painkillers. She has seen two psychologists, a counselor, and a psychiatrist, all of whom thought she was depressed but none knew why it was taking so long for any combination of medication to work. Massage therapy and physiotherapy seemed to help a bit, more so with coping with than with getting rid of pain. Nothing really helped the fatigue. New symptoms arose—forgetfulness, dizziness, clumsiness—and were attributed to the cycle of depression, lack of sleep, fatigue, lethargy, and more depression. It wasn't until she insisted on being tested for lupus that her family doctor ordered a battery of blood tests that could begin to rule out physiological causes for the set of symptoms she was experiencing.

C. E. Multi. Kelp. Calcium-Magnesium. Selenium. Silver. . . . I wonder if I should still be taking silver? . . . Manganese. B_{12}. B_5. . . . "Oh, honey, breakfast looks great." *. . . Hum . . . That should do it. My drops. . . . Where did I put them? . . . They should be . . . here they are. . . . Okay, now. If this won't cure me, nothing will. As if I've not heard that before. . . . Now for the herbs. . . . The water! Don't boil over. Not today! . . . Got it. . . .* "I know it doesn't smell good. But I'm going to drink it anyway." *. . . I wish Danielle could drive. I'm too tired. She could drop me off and I'd let her have the car all day. Sure. Great idea. She'd never remember to pick me up. That's probably not such a good idea. At least it's my short day. That's a pleasant surprise. . . . But now I've got to wait*

for the blood tests until tomorrow. I wonder . . . what they'll say. If anything.
Maybe I've just been on the wrong medication. Or maybe there's a new medica-
tion. There's always something new. . . . I've got to stop this. . . . Okay . . . get
ready for school . . . production, imports, exports . . . trade, tariffs, taxes . . .
what else should a ten-year-old know about the world economy?

After taking a string of pharmaceuticals with little success, Patience looked
further outside the conventional boundaries of healthcare and accessed alternative medicine at the suggestion of a colleague. Sujata assisted Patience in
getting up after a disquieting fall down the steps leading to the front entrance
of the school. The next day during a coffee break she discreetly approached
Patience and asked about the fall. At that time, even though most colleagues
knew she was ill, Patience refused to discuss her state of illness with anyone.
But when Sujata said that naturopathy or homeopathy can be useful in cases
where people are ill for a long time, Patience listened. The major drawback
for such treatment is that the cost is not covered by the provincial health
insurance unless administered by a medical doctor. Sujata suggested a medical doctor who practiced both. Patience went through allergy testing, tinc-
tures, vitamin therapies, and homeopathic remedies. Although vastly
improved, she was only able to increase her paid workload to .5 FTE spread
over four days.

Encouraged by this success, Patience continued to explore alternative
medicine for both diagnosis and treatment. For her birthday last year, her
family got together and purchased her a hair analysis with an iridology exam.
Both tests indicated that she was having troubles with her liver, spleen, and
blood. Though not diagnostic, these alternative ways of conceiving "health"
and "illness" suggested to her that a conventional diagnosis was not just
around the corner. Her family doctor had only recently entertained the idea
that there was a possibility of something other than a psychiatric condition.
For treatment, Patience was able to pursue laser acupuncture for pain management for a limited time as well as reflexology. She was interested in chiro-
practics; however, the number of sessions needed multiplied by the per
session cost was beyond her means. Because of the cost of the naturopathic
and homeopathic supplements, in addition to the increase in cost of weekly
groceries (because of the higher cost of organic food products), Patience had
to choose what types of treatment she could reasonably include on her
income. She found that most alternative treatments were too expensive for
her ongoing use.

So, rather than give up on something that was at the minimum assisting
in maintaining her health/containing her illness, she looked for other lower
priced alternatives. For example, at a recent block party, Patience met Fangni, her new next-door neighbor. During the course of a conversation about
careers, Patience found out that Fangni recently closed her practice as an

acupressure therapist downtown in order to open an alternative health food store servicing the western communities. Fangni had been having difficulties with muscle fatigue and weakness and was finally diagnosed with lupus. She anticipated that shifting from acupressure to retail would help her conserve physical energy and be less wearing on her muscles. As a friendship developed, Patience eventually felt comfortable enough to discuss her chronic symptoms with Fangni, as a friend not as a medical practitioner. Fangni suggested a traditional Chinese herbalist, whom Patience visited for advice. The tea herbs were only $15.00, so she thought she would try it. Though not directly a suggestion, Fangni's experiences of lupus and of the diagnosis process gave Patience enough confidence to ask for the additional blood tests, framed as a request to rule out a disease like lupus.

I wonder if this tea is going to do anything. . . . It doesn't taste as bad as he said it would. . . . What if I'm losing my taste buds. Could that be? I wonder what the doctor would say if I came in with that symptom, too? She would just go back and tell me that I'm depressed and don't want to eat. . . . I already went through this, the weight loss thing. No, I'm not telling her. She wouldn't like that I went to a herbalist anyway. I won't tell her that either. . . . Maybe this doesn't taste so good. Toast. Toast is good. And the melon. This is good. . . . "No, I remember. I'll be there just after school. No problem." *Please don't escalate! I can't take a row this morning. I know I forgot last time. Tuesday. I thought she didn't work today. I'm going to have to ask her write this down for me. . . . I only forgot because . . . I can't remember. She's going to say it. . . .* "I promise. I won't forget this time." *. . . I'm glad I don't have two. Adolescence. Adolescents . . . parents, daughters . . . mothers . . . ill mothers . . . healthy daughters. Me . . . illness . . . me . . . healthy . . .*

1

Setting Out Some Issues

In this book, we offer a feminist materialist analytical framework for understanding and explaining the body. Drawing on feminist theory, critical social geography, critical analyses of women's health, and our own research with women with chronic illness, we propose a radical body politics. For us, a *radical body politics* provides a useful approach in explaining and understanding power and identity through a focus on how both discursive and material aspects of the body shape, mediate, and assist women in negotiating space at a variety of scales. It is a framework that is grounded in and has developed from our work with women with chronic illness and disability, women such as "Patience," introduced in the prologue. Although Patience is fictitious, our description of her and the words we have attributed to her represent a composite of the women from our research. By rethinking the ways in which illness inscribes her body with an ill identity, limits her bodily movements through space, reconstitutes her sense of self, and transforms the minutiae of her daily life, the framework of radical body politics we propose can assist in gaining insight into experiences of body and illness, both hers and of women similar to her. In this sense, Patience acts as a sounding board against which we can toss our ideas about bodies and illness, or even as a conduit for extending theories of identity, power, and space. We must emphasize that integral to our understanding and explanation of Patience's experiences is the sense that these are real women's bodies that we talk about, women who are ill and disabled.

The book then is an exposition of a framework for a radical body politics—one that is feminist, one that draws out discursive formations, one that has a material base, and one that is spatialized. Our framework is radical in that we scrutinize the basis upon which we come to know our social and physical environments and we question the surface meanings of images, texts, and actions. Within the framework, we focus on body, indeed bodies, as both discursive formations and material entities through which we experience those environments. And we describe our framework as a politics because we use our interest in the way power works as an entry point into an extensive understanding and explanation of the process or phenomenon we are investigating, in our case, bodies of women with chronic illness.

Theoretically, we position our work in a literature that brings together critical and feminist analyses of bodies and health. Much of the literature that informs our analysis is interdisciplinary; however, we want to highlight the significance of the contributions of geographers to these discussions as well as show how geographers can enrich feminist critical analyses of body and illness. Indeed, our arguments spill over into other disciplines, taking up some of those debates and reworking concepts to include space. We support this theoretical exposition through empirical illustration from a study carried out in British Columbia, Canada. Although the book draws on one research project we have been working on over the past few years, the framework emerges through information from several projects that focused on the ways in which women use their bodies to structure and restructure their physical and social environments.[1]

Within contemporary feminist and critical social and cultural geography, theoretical and empirical focuses range from various aspects of sexuality and identity, through place-specific activities, to medicalized spaces.[2] Increasingly these works tend to address our embodiment—our *being* through our bodies, whether this be related to sociocultural practices we engage in or to health, illness, and disability.[3] Our proposed framework complements these geographical studies in the sense that we account for physical and social space, the materiality of the body and its discursive construction, and illness and disability by reconceptualizing the everyday experiences of being ill within the context of power and identity. In short, we attempt to *re-embody* women with chronic illness—spatially, materially, discursively, politically—as ill bodies in a healthy society.

FEMINISM, POWER, BODY

With this amplified interest in bodies and spaces in feminist and critical analysis in geography, it seems fitting that our framework be placed more squarely within the interdisciplinary critical literature in feminism on the body, and on illness and disability. Feminist theorists, unsatisfied with conventional notions of the intricacies of power and how it works, turned to poststructuralist accounts of the dispersion of power. And, not surprisingly, analyses of women's bodies changed. With regard to sexual identity, for example, French feminist critiques of psychoanalysis have continually held their ground against the hegemonically dominant reading of Michel Foucault's historical disciplining of the body.[4] But this does not mean that Foucault cannot be useful in understanding women's bodies. By engaging with the Foucauldian concepts of the de-centered subject and a de-centralized power, feminist theorists have challenged fundamentally our ideas about women's bodies and how to approach studying them. In this vein, Judith Butler in *Gender Trouble,* with an extension of this work in *Bodies That Matter,* displaces the notion of sexual difference (including both physiological and biological conceptions) with a performative theory of gender.[5] Butler argues that we act out our gender according to prewritten scripts, scripts that make our actions culturally intelligible. It is through continual performance of cultural scripts of gender that *gendered identities* become stabilized. Although individuals do not, and even cannot, perform *any* gender at *any* given time, they do perform a range of gender that can be understood within their own cultural contexts. Susan Bordo in *Unbearable Weight* and Moira Gatens in *Imaginary Bodies* fashion frameworks that deal sensitively with the cultural and symbolic elements of body construction, respectively.[6] Bordo queries the omnipresence of the image of thinness in Western culture and argues that cultural images associated with body shape homogenize and normalize the self by setting up measures against which women, particularly young women, judge their material bodies. Gatens holds that it is only through analyzing symbolic images of gender and sex, or sexual imaginaries, that we can understand how bodies become part of the wider social and political milieu. Rather than beginning with conventional notions of femaleness and maleness, she maintains that gender itself be understood as sexually, socially, politically, and historically specific. Elizabeth Grosz in *Volatile Bodies* introduces space into her reconfiguration of feminism.[7] She uses space as both an organizational and a conceptual tool to assist her in outlining the corporeality of feminism. She looks at the body from the "inside out" and from the "outside in," distinguishing both the space bodies take up and the space bodies inhabit.

In most feminisms outside poststructuralist literature, analysts routinely feature women's bodies prominently, whether the primary feminist tenets emphasize suffrage, equality, reproduction, equity, difference, or political positioning. Yet because women's bodies have been conceived as both acolytes and shackles, analyses of women's bodies vary widely. For example, Nona Glazer in "Servants to Capital" conceives women's ability to labor as the source of all women's oppression.[8] Such a view understands the body as a site of oppression only because the body can engage in labor. In contrast, Mary O'Brien in *The Politics of Reproduction* reclaims the biological aspects of labor in terms of explaining women's oppression as well as blazing the path to liberation.[9] She posits that men's alienation derives not from being separated from their labor in production as classical Marxist theory would have it; rather, men's alienation arises from their separation of labor in the process of *re*production. We chose these two examples with Felicity Callard's point in mind.[10] She is troubled by the body being primarily theorized in postmodern literature as overlooking, even to the point of dismissing altogether, issues of political economy and Marxist theory. Glazer and O'Brien, writing prior to the explosion of literature on the body, are certainly outside the purview of postmodern theory, yet they still have much to say about women's bodies through their theorizations of the positioning of women's and men's labor within a reformulated political economy.

Feminist geographers have played a central role in the elaboration of spatialized social theories of power.[11] Critical geography's engagement with feminism fuels contributions to social theory, which continues to challenge how power is conceived, how power is deployed, and how to effect social and political change in the context of identity formation.[12] Much critical feminist research in geography, undertaken at a variety of scales, benefits from the analytical insight gained when facing up to this challenge, particularly around themes of identity formation, representation, and difference.[13] Although growing in number, critical feminist accounts within geography have yet to be taken up in all research contexts.

One of these contexts is women's health and illness. Although women's health and illness has had a long acquaintance with feminism, this intersection has not been fully developed in either feminist or health geography. Although common outside health geography, analyses of women's bodies are not all that common within health geography.[14] It is not that health geographers would not welcome and find interesting such a topic with critical perspectives, including feminism; rather, it is more that there has not been a clear agenda for a feminist health studies in geography.[15] It was not until 1994 that Michael Dorn and Glenda Laws invited medical geographers to take seriously both representational and material bodies in their analyses, from which feminists took their direction.[16] Several geographers working in the area of disability as part of health geography are critically engaging these literatures.[17] These studies in disability, however, pose a peculiar incongruity: even though disability is seemingly intrinsically about the body, such studies do not inevitably focus on the body. Because of the dominance of the social model of disability, that emphasizes the social construction of disability through physical and social barriers, it makes sense then that geographical studies in disability do not focus on the body—they focus on the social and physical constraints that prevent disabled bodies and persons with disabilities to participate fully in social life.[18] Furthermore, few geographical studies on disability engage feminist analyses. Again, the introduction of disability studies into geography emanated from a non-feminist, structuralist account of disability. Although arising in response to an individual model of disability, which focused on comparisons of an idealized with disabled (read unabled) bodies, the social model of disability did not take into account the nuances of bodily being that feminism has been able to provide.

THINKING THROUGH THE BODY

In proposing this radical body politics as a way to make sense of women's experiences of illness and the ways in which they negotiate the spaces through which they live, we take up a primary conceptual issue that has been in the forefront of our thinking through the body. In talking with women like Patience, in reading analyses of bodies, in engaging feminist thought, nearly everywhere we turned, we came up against those ever-present dualisms that plague Western thought. Because of our interests in radical body politics, those most prevalent were those that cast the body as either abled or disabled, healthy or ill, normal or deviant. Also salient were those that separated mind from body, truth from fiction, rationality from emotion. Yet the difficulty in dealing with these dualisms is not just that they exist; it is that one side of the dualism is valued over the other—man over woman, culture over nature, health over illness. What is so insidious about dualisms is that they permeate all realms of thought and pose, support, and reproduce a polarized understanding of what it is to exist, to know, and to act. By providing only "either/or" patterns for understanding bodies, dualisms systematically relegate bodily knowledge, as well as the bodies themselves, into multiple sets of binarisms. Bodies cannot exist as *both* abled *and* disabled, healthy *and* ill, normal *and* deviant. Nor are bodies sites where both the mind and body, truth and fiction, rationality and emotion exist together. This centuries-old approach to categorizing and defining knowledge is still prevalent today even with the intricate critiques arising out of postmodern criticism and poststructuralist thought.[19]

Poststructuralists propose alternative ways of understanding the separation of things expressed as dualisms. Two significant critiques arising out of poststructuralism have been Jacques Derrida's discussion of *pharmakon* and Chantal Mouffe's "constitutive outside." Although on quite different topics, these two (cursory) examples provide a glimpse into the ways poststructuralists are making inroads into dislodging the predominance of Western, dualistic thought. Derrida, in "Plato's Pharmacy," uses the Greek term *pharmakon* to frame his discussion of text and writing; *pharmakon* means medicine as a means for healing and/or poison as a means of killing.[20] Taking seriously the premise of ambiguity underlying the construction of the concept of *pharmakon*, wherein categories encompass their own opposites, "either/or" dualisms are shattered, transformed into "either," "or," "both," and "and" choices.

Chantal Mouffe in promoting a radical democratic politics builds on Derrida's notion of the "constitutive outside," wherein vestiges of that which is excluded in the definition of any identity assist in constructing that same identity.[21] With respect to transcending dualisms, Mouffe provides a model whereby the process of setting up dualisms is questioned. Included in any socially constructed identity, whether socially imposed or self-identified, are not just those associations that are taken on willingly, but also those that are rejected outright, including the opposites of that which is incorporated positively into an identity. Thus, the relationship between the sides of a dualism is not mutually exclusive; rather, each side contains parts of the other.

Attempts like these to go beyond the dualisms infusing Western thought saturate the feminist agenda on the body. Whether dealing with theories of women's bodies as essentialist or constructivist or as cultural or biological, feminists claim the need to face the "other" in bodily forms. Implicit in these feminist explanations of the body is the need to undermine other dualisms that influence thinking about the body, not the least of which is the discourse and materiality binary. For feminists working with the body, this is a crucial dualism. With the upsurge in cultural studies throughout the 1980s, interrogating the discursive body, one constructed through text, emerged as the primary way to theorize the body. This is in stark contrast to earlier feminist theory which was primarily located either in matters of biology, with sex as the difference between females and males and gender as the difference between social constructions of femininity and masculinity, or in the materiality of everyday life, with political economy framing the understanding of women's laboring bodies. Approaching the discourse/materiality binary as well as other dualisms in the context of understanding the body for us entails holding in tension the two sides without valuing one over the other, without focusing on one to the detriment of the other. This tension is somewhat like a generic *pharmakon* in that tension describes the relationship between both sides of the binary while circumscribing the two. This tension is also like the "constitutive outside" in that one side of the binary is implicated within the other, and sustains its form and meaning.

CHRONIC ILLNESS, BODY, SPACE

Conceptualizing these dualisms as tensions within a radical body politics can assist in understanding how to make sense of particular configurations of the articulation of power, body, and space. One particular configuration is women's chronically ill bodies, an especially fitting site given how several dualisms play themselves out as women, like Patience, fall ill, seek treatment, adjust to being ill, and form ill identities. Chronic illness is about being both sick and healthy—at the same time. Viewing the body simultaneously as a discursive and material entity while holding discourse and materiality in tension can provide insight into how a woman copes with, treats, and adjusts to living with chronic illness while negotiating what it means to take on an ill identity. Contributions from inside and outside geography have suggested that both discursive and material entities, including bodies, are constituted through space.[22] Some of these same works, in addition to others, have stressed that space is simultaneously both social and physical, without explicitly stating so.[23] Conceiving space simultaneously as a social and physical entity while holding socially constructed, meaning-laden space and the physical layout and contents of space in tension can also provide insight into how a woman with chronic illness deals with being ill and healthy at the same time.

The proposed framework of radical body politics, with the central constructs of body, illness, and environment draws out these tensions associated with experiences of being ill and living with chronic illness. Body is both constituent and conveyor of social, political, and psychological meanings. As well, bodies constitute and are constituted by social relations imbued with power. Yet body is also inscribed variously by biology and physiological processes while simultaneously being constituted through discourse (ideas, notions, texts) and materiality (economy, matter, and substance). Bodies are sites where conceptions of body and bodily experience come together to constitute meaning and corporeality. Illness, too, is constructed through discourse and materiality. Rather than thinking of illness as the presence of disease, or concomitantly health as its absence, we think of illness as simultaneously a category inscribing a body, a physiological process that hinders lust for and the vitality of life, a category constituted by bodily experience, and a process through which identities are shaped. Specific configurations of bodies and illness emerge through both the representations of the material *and* particular materialized discourses (the social practices and specific activities that sustain and reproduce discursive formations). In this way, we can say that we *embody* our everyday experiences. Thus, it is within particular environments that the meanings of those discourses are negotiated—with effects for subjectivities, identities, and spaces.[24] These environments comprise the multiple and varying positions individuals and groups of individuals occupy in the diverse sets of relations they engage—infused with power. Environment in this sense is relational, and certainly not equivalent to space. Space, for us, is both social and physical. It is *lived* experience, *corporeal space*, constituted by and constituting both conceptions and perceptions of space.

WHAT IS CHRONIC ILLNESS?

Showing how this framework can actually be useful in unsettling dualisms, especially that of discourse and materiality, rests on using women's chronically ill bodies to illustrate tension. The first step in such a task is defining what chronic illness is. Chronic illness is readily deemed a long-lasting sickness with no definitive cure on the horizon, a condition of infirmity, a lack of health. Yet describing chronic illness as a long-term sickness does not get at the stuff, the nitty-gritty, that makes chronic illness, chronic illness. Using the descriptor "long-term" doesn't express the intensity of experiencing a specific set of symptoms over a lengthy period of time. Nor does it capture chronic illness as a state of waxing and waning . . . uncertainty . . . indeterminacy . . . fluctuation. This capricious movement inherent in chronic illness sets up individuals to experience both vigor and lethargy, remissions and flare-ups, "good days" and "bad days"—sometimes months apart, sometimes within minutes of each other, sometimes in tandem. For most chronic illness, recurrence of sickness or health is indeterminable. There can be indications of what may or may not exacerbate intensification of symptoms or disease progression, but for the most part chronic illness is laced with uncertainty. These indistinct patterns envelop the everyday life of someone with chronic illness so much so that each detail of life is awash with doubt.

In order to understand, define, and describe the impact of chronic illness on the physical body and daily routines, practitioners and researchers often contrast chronic illness with acute illness and disability. With acute illness, intensity and severity of ill symptoms are short-lived and, as a result, usually respond to immediate intervention. Recovery from acute illness is also shorter and more predictable than recovery from chronic illness. Policy regulating the delivery of health services in North America is oriented toward stabilizing health so that an individual can recover either in an institution or at home. This is a problem for people with chronic illness whose state of health is in flux and the course of disease progression and recovery is unknown. Yet chronic and acute illness are not mutually exclusive. Those with chronic illness can endure acute illness that may complicate the progression of the disease process, as for example, people with lupus developing pneumonia. Onset of chronic illness can follow or even accompany acute illness, as for example, post-viral fatigue syndrome or post-traumatic stress syndrome after an episode of acute illness.

More difficult, however, is the comparison of chronic illness and disability. For example, instead of a focus on the personal limitations of impairment or on the limited capacity of bodily function, the social model of disability calls into question the social organization of society that excludes persons with impairments or impaired bodily functions from mainstream social activities. But what about those with chronic illness whose symptoms are invisible, whose limits on bodily functions fluctuate, whose exclusion is not obvious to either people in the mainstream or disability activists? Defining chronic illness in terms of disability raises questions about which types of illness are disabling and to what extent. Health practitioners, insurance companies, and policymakers are active in setting parameters for designating who is disabled by illness. Homecare policy that limits the delivery of in-home health care services to those people needing personal care, for example, would include persons with disabilities whose needs are for the most part stable and would exclude people with chronic illness whose needs may be more variable. Securing income through public and private insurance may be more difficult for persons with chronic illness than persons with disabilities because of the changeability in the state of illness. People with chronic illness are somewhere between being fully able or completely unable to work—sick-but-fit or fit-but-sick.[25]

This instability is not valued socially in North America, or in many other places where social values are based on attributing worth to one side of a dualism, as for example, *order*/chaos, *linearity*/ non-linearity, *predictability*/ unpredictability, *healthy*/ill, *recoverable illness*/non-recoverable illness. If prevalent views in society are such that chronic illness is seen as part of the "un-worthy" side of the dualism, on the margins, which is indeed a reasonable argument in this context, then what can be gained from speaking from experiences of being chronically ill? From listening to stories of people with chronic illness? bell hooks says that when speaking from the margin (such as the space of chronic illness), one must refuse the center; one must choose the margin as a space of radical openness.[26] To do so would mean unshackling chronic illness from its negative images—from its script of ignominy, lack, disapproval. Does denial and refusal of persons with chronic illness have to do with empathy with persons in pain and suffering or is it about distancing a self from negative sensations and abject bodily forms/constitutions? Is denial and refusal about functioning as "productive" workers? Employees? Mothers? Wives? Daughters? About "pulling one's own weight" in society, economy, and relationships? Is it about not "fitting in" or not permitting the "others" who are "different" to "fit in"? Is it a fear of abnormality? Of deviance? Of death? Of dying? Is it a rejection of difference? Is it about seeing the margins from the center? In order to refuse the center and choose the margin, women with chronic illness could possibly claim their body not as an illness or even a site of illness, but *as a body in an ill society.* For it is only when unpredictability, instability, and unsteadiness are valued that persons with chronic illness can no longer be seen as "different." They would just be/come.[27]

WHAT IS TO COME

This description of chronic illness sets up the discussion comprising the rest of the book. In this chapter, we set out issues we take up in the following chapters. We first presented a proposal for a radical body politics, one that is feminist, one that draws out discursive formations, and one that has a material base, one that is spatialized. We located our project at the intersection of poststructuralist conceptions of power, feminist theory, critical social geography, and women's experiences of chronic illness. We make the case that thinking through the body entails challenging the dualisms inherent in Western thought. By conceiving dualisms, not as mutually exclusive entities, but as tensions within and between both sides of binary constructions, we propose to interrogate a particular configuration of power, body, and space—women's chronically ill bodies. Once we understand women's bodies as simultaneously discursive and material entities and space as both social and physical, then we can use a radical body politics to make sense of women's experiences of illness, women much like Patience.

In chapter 2, we provide a background from which our project emerged, that is, we review literature that has influenced our thinking about the body, identity, women's health, and space. In chapters 3 and 4, we detail the framework we are proposing for a radical body politics in preparation for the empirical illustrations. We organize this exposition around a set of concepts we find useful: discourse, materiality, power, spatiality, embodiment, and corporeal space. In chapter 5, we discuss some of the methodological issues we faced while undertaking these projects and provide a description of the women whose experiences we draw on to demonstrate our arguments. Our empirical material illustrating our proposed radical body politics comprises the following four chapters—discourse (chapter 6), materiality (chapter 7), identity (chapter 8), and spatiality (chapter 9). Finally, in chapter 10, we rethink our framework, reconnect issues that have framed our presentation, and revisit themes we have identified as important along the way.

2

❧

Working through Theories of the Body

For the past decade, there is no doubt that the body has played the starring role in feminist theory. Leading the way have been works in philosophy, sociology, and cultural studies.[1] In geography, too, there has been a marked increase in interest in the body.[2] It makes sense that in an age of late capitalism where images of bodies dominate visual media—magazines, television, Internet—that interest would increase in how these ideal, contrived, and/or fantasy bodies affect real, tangible, physical bodies. For women, having a hegemonically defined "beautiful" body often translates into increased self-confidence and sexual assuredness. What that beautiful white[3] body looks like is increasingly being tied to healthy, lean, svelte, "fit" bodies.[4] In order to achieve "success," women are turning not only to healthier foods, natural skin care products, and cosmetic surgery, but also to more intense bodily activities like body building and rigorous fitness regimes.[5]

There is no doubt that the proliferation of popular(ized) images of beautiful bodies has contributed to the intellectual appeal of theorizing the body. Images of bodies, however, are not the only impetus feeding the frenzy for feminists' choices to theorize the body. It also makes sense that in an age where physical bodies appear to be endless—through population growth, reproductive technologies, cloning—that interest would swell in figuring out how "scientific knowledge" can affect physical bodies. The complete mapping of human DNA and the use of stem cell growth to repair organs are two biomedical technologies that have the potential to transform not only how we understand physiological and biological processes of the body but also how bodies themselves are created.[6] Yet alongside these so-called advances in medicine, the fragility and imperfection of the body has once again emerged as something to ponder, especially in the face of unpredictable

19

outbreaks of deadly viruses such as Ebola, necrotizing fasciitis, and HIV.[7] Such certainty around processes of creation linked with uncertainty around destructive forces creates a collective cultural angst about technology, and thus inquiries into the ability of the human body to survive intact throughout the twenty-first century through, for example, delaying "old age."[8]

Augmenting these empirical reasons for an increasing interest in theorizing the body is the concomitant widespread turn to subjectivity in social theory. This turn, too, makes sense in that the body is a "logical" place to investigate subjectivity and identity for this is the site through which people experience life. Once focused on the body as a site to investigate subjectivity, a plethora of other topics associated with identity spring forward and call for attention—subject positions, gender as performativity, articulation of power relations, and autobiography as personal criticism.[9] Through these active theorizations, body has not only come to be associated with individual subjectivities; body has become the site through which to sort society.[10]

Thinking through theories of the body, including notions of being different, ill, disabled, and deviant, shaped our project. Throughout our engagement with this work, we have always been drawn to two types of theorists. One group focuses on how women's identities emerge through prevailing ideas about how the body *should* be—whether these ideas be about work, sexuality, or body shape. This led us to an interest in how women are empowered to resist these prevailing ideas and actively pursue identities seemingly alternative to the hegemonic ones so prevalent in women's everyday lives. Refusing prescriptive notions of body, including, for example, body images based on fads, fashion, or fitness, and replacing them with sets of non-prescriptive sets of ideas, unsettles the dominance of one particular(ized) body—even in counterhegemonic circles.[11] Another group comprises those theorists that attempt to deal with the biological aspects of the body, in terms of sexuality as well as bodily form. This emphasis on the palpability of bodies, their substance, made us think about how women use their bodies and their experiences of their bodies to structure and restructure the spaces they inhabit daily. Accounting for the alteration of surrounding spaces to accommodate bodily form and function reinstates bodily existence as both an entity unto itself and a part of a spatialized context—socially, physically, politically, economically, and culturally. Together these theoretical works have invited us to think through some fundamental dualisms surrounding inquiries into the body.

In this chapter, we first work through some attempts at categorizing theories of the body to show how thinking about the body has affected the way we approach our understanding of women's experiences of chronic illness. We then review some of the theoretical works about the body that have influenced our radical body politics, paying close attention to feminist accounts of psychoanalytic theory, discourse, and identity. We close by indicating the way we have chosen to approach theorizing ill bodies in our radical body politics.

CATEGORIZING THEORIES OF THE BODY

Categorizing approaches to theorizing the body is useful when trying to sort through the interaction between discursive categories and the material body. Analysts suggesting ways to categorize theory tend to provide schemes that reflect their underlying epistemological claims. Anne Witz makes a similar point when she argues that the corporealization of bodies in sociological theory has been premised on the idea that men have comprised the social and women have always been part of the corporeal.[12] Thus, "bringing the body back in" is not about focusing on bodies; rather, it is about focusing on those bodies that have been absent. Our concern here, unlike Witz who was interested solely in gender, is about the discursive and the material and how each are represented in theories of the body. To this end, we review three categorizations of theories—suggested by Chris Shilling, Elizabeth Grosz, and Simon Williams and Gillian Bendelow—to show the passage from modernist notions of arranging bodies according to dualistic categories toward postmodern ones that draw attention to bodily variation as a state of being, and onward toward ones that attempt to break away from dualistic thinking altogether.

Chris Shilling distinguishes between naturalistic and social constructionist approaches.[13] Naturalistic approaches conceive the body as a biological entity upon which social norms and values are attached and layered. Feminisms that emphasize the reproductive capacity of females as the source of male oppression can be considered naturalistic. In creating explanations of social and political oppression, such theorists would link oppressive acts to the biological makeup of women, such as the capacity to give life, or to physiological processes that are part of reproduction, such as lactation, menses, or hormonal fluctuations. These types of approaches have been widely criticized for defining too narrowly causal relationships between behavior and biology, being too deterministic in not permitting individual agency, and confining too restrictively the notion of oppression. Social constructionist approaches conceptualize the body as the product of social interaction. Feminisms that emphasize such a recursive relationship focus on discursive constructions that constrain, shape, or create the body, such as the beautiful body or the slender body. Explanations of social and political oppression tend to see the body as both the problem and the solution. Critics point out that these types of approaches do not take seriously the non-discursive elements in society and polity. This refusal to incorporate material aspects of the body leaves bodies untouchable, suspended in text, outside the purview of daily life, everyday living.

Shilling argues that it is important to incorporate both the natural body and the socially constructed body into a theory that seeks to explain how the body interacts with and in society. Because most people are aware of the transformative potential that intervention in natural bodily processes has to alter the body, especially through surgery and drugs, the notion of the ideal body and its attainment through crucial lifestyle choices persists. Yet the high cost of such interventions severely restricts access to those without the corresponding means. He argues that a site ripe for exploring both aspects is the body in transition, going from one state of being into another; the socially constructed body highlights the unfinished nature of a body that is shaped by life choices and the natural body can account for bodily existence. Shilling focuses on the dying body because this site of transition—from life to death—accentuates the entwinement of the natural and socially constructed body. The physiological process of death extinguishes the natural body and its intricate biology. And, while dying, people are embroiled in the social organization of death—emotionally, culturally, economically, socially, and existentially.

Shilling's argument here can be useful for understanding what women with chronic illness face once they become ill. For example, women with chronic illness are in a state of transition—from health to illness. And, because of ever-changing symptoms, the transition itself fluctuates—from illness to a good day to relative illness to health to more health to a bad day to more illness to. . . . However, unlike death, there is not necessarily a termination of bodily existence. Thus, what is frustrating is that the expectations of bodily intervention to alter the body favorably through drugs, therapies, and lifestyle changes often fail, leaving women with aspirations of an idyllic, healthy body without a well-trodden path to reach that ideal. As a result, women with chronic illness live a tumultuous, chaotic existence through which the natural and socially constructed bodies are often indistinguishable, yet incongruent—although discursively ill, there may be no obvious symptoms or there may be symptoms that do not "fit" the specific category of chronic illness. Women must negotiate the social organization of illness, made manifest through biomedical practitioners (doctors, therapists), social networks (friends, family), and financial organizations (benefits analysts, insurance adjusters), in order to make themselves culturally intelligible as women with chronic illness.

Shilling's categorization is helpful in understanding transition. However, we are cautious about pursuing a seemingly simplistic merging of natural and socially constructed bodies in "high" modernity for two reasons. First, the project of the body is defined in terms of a society comprised of many individual bodies. To emphasize any particular(ized) body, a chronically ill female body included, seems rather artificial in light of the complexities of bodily living. Any such distinction seems to proclaim the fit between bodies and society as the central theme in the overall project rather than constitution of society, polity, and economy *through* bodies. Second, this merging perpetuates the separation of mind and body in the theorization of the body. Distilling experience, such as the existential angst of being within the context of social regulation, to one of an unmediated state of being does not consider seriously the complexities arising from social and cultural relations and interaction. Figuring out how and under what circumstances the socially constructed body or the natural body is both constraining and enabling glosses over what the unique sensuality of bodily existence has to offer theory.

Another approach to categorizing theory about the body, perhaps more attuned to thinking about chronically ill bodies, noted by Elizabeth Grosz, differentiates between the "inscriptive" and "lived" bodies.

> The first conceives the body as a surface on which social law, morality, and values are inscribed; the second refers largely to the lived experience of the body, the body's internal or psychic inscription. Where the first analyzes a *social*, public body, the second takes the body-schema or imaginary anatomy as its objects(s).[14]

Surface, or *external*, bodily inscriptions include those material manifestations of social, cultural, and political ideas, notions, and thoughts about the body. Stiletto heels, makeup, and breast implants are all obvious examples of the ways in which women in North America culturally modify their bodies in accordance to hegemonic notions of beauty. Other inscriptions are not so obvious. For example, a 1999 ruling by the Supreme Court of Canada designated that the sexual histories of sexual assault victims are not permitted to be included as part of the defense of the person being tried for sexual assault. This act inscribes the sexually violated body as pristine, in a sense, one that is unconnected to previous sexual behavior. This uncoupling of ongoing sexual behavior and the act of sexual assault reinstates[15] the sexually violated body as a separate entity, underscoring the movement toward accepting that when a woman says no, she means no. Psychic, or *internal*, inscriptions include those meanings of body and bodily functions that are actively incorporated into a child's notion of body. It is not that these inscriptions are generated internally; rather, the body is always already coded, particularly sexually, so that a child's notion of body emerges through cultural signification processes of sexual difference. With these approaches, women's bodies are contrasted with males and subsequently conceptualized as castrated, lacking, and incomplete.[16] Either way—through external or internal inscription—the body is still a site that can be "read" or made culturally intelligible.

Grosz's differentiation between the two types of inscription acts as a way to categorize theory of the body about the body—those theories that see the body as a surface to inscribe and those that see the body as a generator of its own inscriptions. Like Grosz, we do not think that reconciliation between the two bodies is possible; for us, it would not even be desirable. The two extremes of her external and internal inscriptive bodily surfaces set up an irreconcilable dichotomy. Conceiving the body as a surface upon which culture is layered reduces the body to a passive vessel, void of any interactive capacity—neither actively constructive, nor inertly complicit. Conceiving the body as already and always coded, particularly sexually, not only privileges the sexed body over other bodies, but also diminishes the importance of multiple cultural coding systems. Yet Grosz's distinction is still useful when thinking about women's chronically ill bodies because the process through which bodies become marked for cultural intelligibility can be traced. Discourse about chronic illness does matter when dealing with the variety of institutions women with chronic illness have to deal with—hospitals, workplaces, insurance companies, and government—especially with regard to the words used to describe symptoms and the disease itself. Even though sexual difference is indeed prominent in understanding sensual experiences, so too are other sensorial and emotional experiences, like that of pain, fatigue, malaise, and frustration, sadness, relief.

Simon Williams and Gillian Bendelow provide yet another categorization of theories about the body, at least indirectly.[17] Their project consists of critically re-reading writings on the body in both classical and contemporary sociological writings and differentiating a *sociology of the body* from an *embodied sociology*. They organize their framing discussion around two themes arising from the relationship between body and society, and, as a result, categorize theories of the body according to those that stress bodily "order"[18] and those that emphasize bodily "control."[19] Such a typology avoids long-standing disputes over sociology and biology and somewhat shadows structure-agency debates. Theories of bodily "order" attempt to explain the regulation and restriction of individual bodies socially, as for example, through etiquette, rituals, and ceremonies. Theories of "control" focus on how individuals influence and choose to live their lives as well as how they express themselves in social interaction, as for example, through gaining access to change and resisting dominating power relations.

This sorting of social theories of the body is what Williams and Bendelow call the "sociology of the body": descriptions and analyses of various and multiple bodies in offering explanations of individual behavior in light of bodily existence and interaction. What they prefer are theories that can directly address bodily routines, bodily activities, and bodily sensations as well as respect the knowledge immanent within the body. They provide critical overviews of work on and about *real* bodies—female bodies, sleeping bodies, "high" modernity bodies, emotional bodies, painful bodies, and performing bodies. Through each overview, they argue that these somewhat neglected bodies are fertile sites for fostering a truly *embodied* sociological theory—theory that "treats the bodily basis of social order and action as central, and takes the embodiment of its practitioners as well as its subjects seriously."[20] Their point is to encourage theorizing "*from*' lived bodies."[21] For example, conceiving pain as a bodily sensation and an emotional state of being, both with socially mediated meanings, may produce theory that is outside the conventional binarisms that circumscribe pain in "high" modern society—mind/body, reason/emotion, culture/nature. Relocating pain at the intersection of mind, body, and culture (and perhaps even reason, emotion, and nature) loosens the hold of the dominant view of pain as a "controllable" bodily sensation.[22] Once loosened, the notion of pain-free existence dissipates, paving the way to a more holistic understanding, explanation, and experience of pain.

Conceptually, rather than merging socially constructed and natural approaches to explanations of the body (à la Shilling) or reconciling inscriptive and lived bodies (à la Grosz), Williams and Bendelow propose going *through* dualisms. Repositioning concepts like pain, sleep, feelings, and death along competing sides of traditional dualisms breaks apart binary thinking and permits theory to emerge from the messy world of everyday living. For women with chronic illness, this might be a more useful approach because of the flexibility in linking ideas to experiences, feelings, and bodily sensations. Because of the undulating rhythms of their ill bodies, women with chronic illness fail to adhere to the tightly fixed conceptual binary world of "high" modernity. Their varied, multiple, and contradictory experiences of being ill, obtaining a diagnosis, and searching for legitimacy as an ill person fundamentally challenges cultural meanings of being ill, the social organization of illness, and perhaps even definitions of illness itself.

WHAT TO KEEP AND WHAT TO THROW AWAY

From these typologies, it is easy to get a sense that theories on/about/through the body tend to address some aspect of the materiality of the body or discourse about the body, whether highlighting bodily being, acting, or meaning. Yet none of the types of theories discussed breaks apart the dualism of discourse and materiality, at least not to our satisfaction. Most theories, as Shilling notes, tend to privilege either the biological and natural over the representational and intangible aspects of the body or vice versa. Getting outside these dualisms is difficult indeed, for even Shilling's categorization itself reproduces the same dichotomy between the "social"/discourse and "natural"/materiality. Creating theory that incorporates both without privileging one over the other could further open up understandings of the body because, as Grosz points out, material bodies exist as both the entities through which the discursive manifests as well as the physical container (and conveyor) of bodily experiences, which are always already coded. Yet Grosz, too, seems to reproduce a similar set of binaries in her discussion of inscriptions ("external"/discourse and "internal"/materiality) and, to a lesser extent, of lived bodies.[23] So, as we organized our arguments about women, body, and illness around the act of shattering dualisms and binary thinking, we came to realize that "shattering" was something beyond our capabilities, and have chosen instead an unsettling path of destabilization, much like Williams and Bendelow did in their critical re-reading of body theories. As a way around this conundrum, Williams and Bendelow sought to theorize bodies in their entirety, *as they are* and *from how they are*. Likewise, rather than take on the destruction of the dualisms of man/woman, mind/body, and health/illness, we chose instead the binary of discourse and materiality as the focal point of our project. With this focus, we can interrogate the subjugated sides of the dualisms—women, body, illness—as part of a radical body politics that can destabilize unitary and monolithic categories as well as account for destabilizations of material bodies through, for example, the onset of illness and subsequent changes in daily living that help the women restructure their living environments. We locate our attempt to theorize the body at the nexus of women, body, and illness so that we can loosen the connections between discourse and materiality and begin the task of disentangling how it is that bodies are constituted discursively and materially. Exposing the history of the formation of our ideas can only be accomplished by recalling some of what we decided to keep and some of what we decided to throw away.

Feminist writings on the body span several disciplines, as diverse as literary criticism, nursing, and theology.[24] For our project, we have paid close attention to writings that conceive bodies as both discursive constructs and as corporeal entities, and that attempt to thwart the dualism of discourse and materiality, mostly in the fields of sociology, philosophy, anthropology, and geography. Our interest in reading these depictions of bodies intensified as we sought to understand and explain experiences of women with chronic illness. Our engagement with this literature alongside our reading of the women's accounts have profoundly shaped our analysis and interpretation presented in chapters 6, 7, 8, and 9. Three sets of works about the body and identity have influenced our thinking about the articulation of discourse and materiality: feminist incarnations of psychoanalysis, feminist applications of Michel Foucault's work on the body, and feminist elaborations of identity.[25]

Feminist incarnations of psychoanalysis have, as Elizabeth Grosz argues,

> enabled feminists and others to reclaim the body from the realms of immanence and biology in order to see it as a psycho-social product, open to transformations in meaning and functioning, capable of being contested and re-

signified. Feminists have stressed that the generic category "*the* body" is a masculinist illusion. There are only concrete bodies, bodies in the plural, bodies with a specific sex and color. This counterbalances psychoanalysis's tendency to phallocentrism, especially the ways it understands the female body. If the female body is castrated, this is not, contrary to Freud, simply a matter of seeing. Rather, we learn how to see and understand according to prevailing systems of meaning and value, not nature. If the body is plastic, malleable and amenable to social re-inscription, this means that the female body is *a priori* capable of being seen and understood outside the notion of castrated privation. This is only one of a number of possible meanings, but the very one men and women have up to now had little possibility of refusing.[26]

Although her claims are wide and sweeping, Grosz indicates the range of contributions that feminists engaging psychoanalytic theory have to offer, something that cannot be ignored. There is no doubt that psychoanalysis has been important in destabilizing "the body" to include bodies—concrete ones. This scrutiny of specific bodies has called into question the process through which bodies become marked as *specific* bodies. Many postmodern and poststructural accounts of specific bodies show how various set of power relations work together to reproduce the masculine norms of universality and neutrality.[27] Through this reproductive process, some groups become "more universal" than others with the white, heterosexual, male, abled bodies of all ages at the pinnacle. Understanding how specific bodies relate to the "outside" world, in reference to the world outside the immediacy of the material body, has been useful in figuring out the constitutive processes of self, subjectivity, and identity.[28]

There are some difficulties with psychoanalytic accounts of the formation of self, subjectivity, and identity. Much of the postmodern project engages the modern humanist tradition and feminists using poststructural tenets tend to locate their arguments in this intellectual context.[29] When coupling deconstruction as a method for accessing the cultural with psychoanalytic theory, feminists engaging poststructuralism have tended to concentrate on language, signs, and meanings of, particularly, sex and gender. Often in the detailing of basic arguments, theory becomes so abstract that everyday life and the concreteness of specific bodies become lost in a series of claims and assertions. Theory describes what may be going on in abstract terms, but sometimes fails to extend how these abstractions actually come together to constitute the self, the body, and identity in ways that matter in understanding and explaining everyday life. This loss in the process of translating the abstract into the concrete troubles us because, although sympathetic to the arguments, we are left without theory that can assist us in understanding and explaining how women with chronic illness live their daily lives.

Two works have been especially influential for us in working through critiques of psychoanalytic theory: Judith Butler's *Gender Trouble* and Jana

Sawicki's *Disciplining Foucault*.[30] Both draw extensively on Michel Foucault's theories of the body and the self, especially as they have been elaborated in *Discipline and Punish, History of Sexuality: An Introduction, Volume 1*, and *History of Sexuality: The Care of the Self, Volume 3*.[31] Judith Butler criticized feminist work using psychoanalytic theory, especially Julia Kristeva and Luce Irigaray's works, as being too far-reaching and universalist in tenor. She maintains that feminists should explore masculinist totalizing tendencies while at the same time be self-critical of their own.[32] Her project is to dissolve the notion of fixity of identity, particularly gender identities, and replace it with a notion more flexible, variable, and subversive. In the pursuit of recasting gender without the deterministic links of biology, she argues that feminists need, too, to toss aside any notion of a gendered core revolving around any type of essence.[33] She draws on Foucault's project of theorizing the body to develop a performative theory of gender, one where gender constitutes the identity it purports to be.[34] Reformulating the basis upon which the subject is conceived necessarily subverts traditional accounts of identity. She argues that this deconstruction of identity is not the end of politics; rather, the political is opened up at the very points where identities are articulated.[35]

Jana Sawicki is much harsher in her criticisms and dismisses feminist analyses using psychoanalytic theory, declaring that Kristeva and Irigaray offer only three options: to speak in a masculine voice, to construct a new language, or to be silent—none of which is an option for feminists.[36] She makes the point that instead of either legitimating or reformulating psychoanalytic concepts, such as castration or lack, feminists should be looking at the normalizing tendencies within psychoanalysis and conceiving these as dangers. What matters then is the deployment of discourse for all discourses have the potential to be dangerous. Discourses, including psychoanalytic theory and others, can only be designated as either oppressive or liberating in a historical sense and not merely by proclamation.[37] Feminists need to be vigilant about figuring out when a particular discourse or theory is used as a tool of oppression or domination and be able to act accordingly. Resistance, as Sawicki argues in extension of Foucault's notion of power, is possible within limits and should not be judged according to the level of success.[38] With this resistance comes a plurality of possible politics—ones that include diverse "selves," unfixed subjectivities, and a multiplicity of identities.[39]

Like Butler and Sawicki, we do not accept psychoanalytic theory's universalizing and normalizing claims and agree that feminist theoretical accounts need to be self-critical. We also think that identities are unfixed, even fluctuating, giving rise to a wide range of possibilities for politics—ones that are not inherently conservative, liberal, or radical, emancipatory or oppressive. Yet these works, and works like them, remain troubling to us in ways that are difficult to express because our objections themselves are unfixed, fleeting, and in flux.[40] In some instances, explaining individual and collective identities in terms of "performing gender" makes sense and provides insights that can be used when thinking about other *specific* bodies.[41] In other accounts, drawing on psychoanalytic theory seems only to confuse the issue by setting up a straw figure to critique so as to promote psychoanalysis as the most appropriate way to be feminist. Even though we may agree with the point being made, we do not agree with the manner in which some authors substantiate their argument. For us, it is a matter of engaging psychoanalytic theory *critically* just like any other theoretical tradition we might draw on rather than promoting it as a panacea.

For this project, we prefer to highlight the deconstruction of the binary of discourse and materiality, and focus on how this translates into a radical body politics. To illustrate the point we are making, we have chosen to critique Elspeth Probyn's work on sexing the self.[42] Her work exemplifies a way of engaging critically with a plethora of theories about self in order to highlight her own claims about gendered selves and identities. For example, Probyn comes to her own conceptualization of self through engaging in the work of several male, humanist anthropologists interested in the notion of self—Clifford Geertz, James Clifford, George Marcus, and Michael Fisher among others—after she has already problematized the notion of the feminine through feminists using psychoanalytic theory—Monique Wittig, Alice Jardine, and Marilouise and Arthur Kroker. To further her analysis, she engages her own thoughts about the self through Michel Foucault's notions of self and body.[43] By doing so, Probyn is able to reassess critically her own engagement with theory—as a female and as a feminist.[44] She both embraces and maintains a critical distance with some of Foucault's notions and concepts as well as the psychoanalytic feminine self. In her quest to explain experience beyond the individual, Probyn seeks to find a point of articulation between experience and self. She theorizes self as a speaking position,

> This is to say that the self spoken invokes a particular moment of being, but that in its speaking it demands an acknowledgment of the conditions of its possibility, of its very existence. Quite simply, the sound of its "ontologicality" must be met with an analysis of the positivity of its materiality. This is not to "recognize the self in its otherness," but always to ask what had to be in place in order for this self to appear at all. Rather than embracing the other as a discursive relation wherein she disappears into the same, this self is an acutely self-conscious entity; her speech makes me feel strange. I should be clear here that I am not suggesting that we all remake ourselves as "exotic," or as an undifferentiated equivalence of others among others; rather, I want to posit a self as a speaking position that entails a defamiliarization of the taken-for-granted. It is a speaking position that . . . is firmly based in an epistemological questioning of how it is that I am speaking. Speaking my self thus should render me uneasy in my skin, *pas bien dans ma peau*, as it decentralizes any assurance of ontological importance.[45]

How we interpret what she is saying about self is that instead of being defined through boundaries set in relation to an "other" or through "lack," speaking the self is a conscious entity that articulates her ontological status deliberately and knowingly. The self is no longer based on differentiating "I" from "you," "her," "him," "we," or "they"; rather, the self is stripped of its familiar status located in everyday existence and speaks without any pre-set, pre-assumed, or pre-determined positioning. The conditions of possibility include both experience and the politicization of experience. Theoretically, then, according to Probyn, the speaking self is unattached to individuals and concrete bodies while at the same time being rooted in the specifics of her own local materiality.

> [T]he self both expresses the specificities of local power relations and allows us to figure them in ways that can be analyzed. In that the self is seen as both practice and the problematization of practices, the investigation of power struggles and relations is undertaken through the self, thus ensuring that the analysis is both historical and reflective of the given situation. It is a self conceived of as within the force of a critical attitude.[46]

Through this "critical attitude," the self makes choices about how to engage the world and becomes a way to think, feel, and act.[47]

We think that the process through which Probyn develops her arguments is indeed superb. Yet in the end her conceptualization of self falls apart when materialized. Probyn acknowledges that speaking the self tends to become synonymous with "I" and the individual, as she expressed as speaking "my self."[48] In order to move beyond this inward exclusion, she links everyday experience to the imagination. She considers the articulation as *imagined space,* a place where individuals—situated along various axes of power—are acknowledged and set aside so that interaction can take place equitably and justly. Unfortunately, what Probyn fails to consider in this imagined space, perhaps because imagined spaces are by definition idyllic, is the complexity of the materiality of self. She remains suspended in a theoretical discourse on the self that she herself assisted in creating. The problem is that once real interaction takes place, the delicate balance is upset and the interaction cannot be equitable or just *precisely because the personal material histories of the actors and of the (political, cultural, economic) moment flood the space.*

In Probyn's own example of how speaking selves work in action, she notes that feminists as speaking subjects are continually hemmed into having to speak about what they consider to be basic notions, claims, and politics. After having been seduced into the speaking position offered, as a feminist talking about the backlash against political correctness within universities in her example, she experiences the space open to her for speaking as limited, serving only to displace what really is needed to be said.[49] Because of her focus on the subject as a speaking position, she does not give enough attention to how selves are arranged in relationship to one another—not in the sense of defining self as "not other" but in the sense of a space where multiple selves necessarily have to exist. In her example of speaking selves, she seems to privilege what we know about our "selves" (read singularly, as many "myselves") over the experiences of "our" selves (read as the collective, or many "selves"). Pushing Probyn's analysis a littler further, it seems to us that self, even if situated along the surface between being and knowing as Probyn claims, needs to be materialized not only through attitude but through positioning with multiple selves. In engaging those relations, the self shifts as a speaking position to yet another speaking position, to another, and still another. The self continually reemerges through our selves in relation to one another. We would call this the experience of maneuvering through daily life in order to find out who "I am" and who "we are."

In works relying on psychoanalytical theory, Probyn included, we think that discourse is being privileged over materiality. Granted, works using Foucault's anti-humanist exegesis of the self and body would tend to focus on discourse, for it is his notion of discourse that sent ripples throughout the academy: discourse is both the structure of language *and* the materiality of the social practices that sustain it.[50] Yet these works still elide the material in favor of elaborating the discursive via focusing on developing arguments pertaining to persons performing an abstract construct (like gender with Butler), destabilizing dogmatic politics (like resistance with Sawicki), and materializing identity through imagination (like self as a speaking position with Probyn). This is not to say that these types of works are not useful in understanding the body discursively or materially. Analyses of bodily discourse demonstrate quite clearly how it is that abstractions, such as language, ideas, and text about the body, define the parameters of and give meaning to the body.[51] But problems arise when identity and positionings within webs of power are not made concrete as part the materiality of the bodily discourse.[52] Emergence of identity in specific places is fraught with difficulties in figuring out what matters most at any given time—ability, age, class, ethnicity, race, sex, or sexuality—even though feminists know politically that ranking oppressions and privileging specific identities is not always useful and can be dangerous.[53]

Elaborating identity outside the masculinist pattern of establishing hierarchies has been a major endeavor for feminists throughout the past two decades. Figuring out how identity emerges, individually and collectively, through the body has dominated feminist elaborations of identity with regard to gender, sexuality, race, and class.[54] One important contribution feminists have made to the discussions of identity formation or constitution is that biological make up, expressions of sexuality, skin color, and status of labor are not distinguishing features of identity; the social, cultural, eco-

nomic, and political meanings ascribed to each comprise the source for differentiation and valuing in dualistic Western thought. Examining states of
being, knowing, and acting have been useful in sorting through those processes through which bodies take on and project meaning, multiple meanings. Theorizations of identity have played out, for example, as identity
theorized as social differentiation, as an intersection of social locations, or as
integral to cultural intelligibility.[55] One of the drawbacks, as Probyn has
already noted, is that studies about self, subjectivity, and indeed identity tend
to focus on the individual, often to the detriment of groups of individuals.[56]
Another drawback to such a focus on identity is that, when conceived as part
of the modern project, identity is nearly always framed by a discussion of
sameness and difference. Chantal Mouffe, as we discussed in chapter 1, uses
the "constitutive outside" to explain the relationship between self and other
(corresponding to sameness and difference).[57] In more detail, her argument
rests on two basic premises: (1) any identity of a "we" is based on excluding
some "other" and (2) subject positions are constituted through sets of social
relations. When thinking about how "self" and "other" are (re)produced,
Mouffe points out that the processes are closely entwined—within any identity of "I" there is always some remnant of that which is being excluded, the
"other," even if it is only through absence. As any identity is being constituted, there is already an inclusion in some form of the "outside," already an
imbrication of "other" with "I." Conceived in this way, no identity is complete, permanent, or singular for there is always already present both that
which is and that which is not. Mouffe goes on to argue that because identities are constituted through various and multiple sets of social relations, there
is no *specific* identity that cannot be resisted, because there is no self-referen-
tial point that is outside the process of constitution.

In the context of connecting *specific* identities as a strategy for creating a
"we," Mouffe claims that this slipperiness of non-closure of identity means
that there is no definitive or predetermined link to or with other people.
Any connection forged through any set of social relations is fleeting and in
flux. Yet this does not mean that there is no basis for collective identity or
groups of people with similar interests, attributes, or desires. She uses the
concept of *nodal point* to describe temporary fixations around which identities coalesce. Nodal points result from hegemonic processes through which
identities come to be conceived as tightly defined, fixed, and natural. Disrupting these nodal points can help in transforming identities from a static,
politically immobile set of associations to a dynamic, politically mobilizing
set. Mouffe's theory of the way through which individual identities can join
together to create collective identities is useful in understanding the experiences of women with chronic illness. She says that even though identities are
fluctuating, indeterminate, and conditional, they can become fixed through
the ways power is deployed in society, discursively and materially.

Mouffe's use of the concepts "constitutive outside" and "nodal point" might be helpful in understanding identities that have been marginalized within theoretical discourses on identity and difference, as for example, that of bisexual identities and community. Bisexual identities are not comfortably located in conjunction with either heterosexual or homosexual identities, politics, or communities, nor in resistance to heterosexuality or homosexuality. Bisexuals are both heterosexual and homosexual, and neither at the same time. Attempts to locate bisexual theorizing in a sea of queer and feminist theory ultimately fail because of the way in which feminists and queer theorists have engaged bisexuality theoretically in terms of sameness and difference.[58] In a Western, dualistic world where *A* or *not A* define the parameters of who "I" and who "she" is, it is no small wonder that those who are *both* *A* and *not A* cannot find a comfortable place theoretically or empirically, discursively or materially. Perhaps an emergent nodal point for a *specific* identity (associated with a *specific* body) is bisexuality, which is momentarily fixed but still unstable enough to be rearticulated with other identities to form other collective identities as nodal points.[59]

Theorizing community, too, poses a similar problem. Community, most commonly understood as a group of people with some similarity, whether it be, for example, geographical, political, or sexual similarity, falls apart when the community grows and becomes more diverse. Encompassing this diversity while pursuing some unified identity is precisely what is at issue. Iris Marion Young challenges the notion of this "ideal community" and offers the unoppressive city as open to unassimilated otherness.[60] Her competing conceptualization implies an inexhaustibility of the possibilities of articulations among diverse persons, spaces, and groups of people. By coupling Mouffe's notion of nodal points with Young's concept of the unoppressive city, the fluidity and conditionality of identities can be maintained without sacrificing any one specific identity for any other.

We cite these two examples because of the loose but significant parallels we see between them and women with chronic illness. Like bisexuals, women with chronic illness are "in between" hegemonic discourses—not quite ill but not quite healthy, almost disabled and almost abled, both very nearly normal and very nearly deviant.[61] This positioning has theoretical and political implications. Theoretically, acknowledging that there exists something in between oppositional constructs paves the way for resisting and destabilizing dualisms inherent in Western thinking. Politically, women with chronic illness struggle to claim a(n identity) position that would "make sense" within social relations already constituted/constituting various identities. This latter point leads us to our second example, that of community. Women with chronic illness can illustrate the point that Young makes about the unoppressive city—women with chronic illness as a variable amalgamation of *specific* bodies are unassimilated others, existing at the interstices of *specific* identities.

They destabilize the notions of sameness and difference because within the amalgamation of *specific* bodies there exist no normative notions of health or of illness; it is only when these women engage medical, financial, and paid work discourses to take on a regime of treatment, secure an income, or go on sick leave that specific definitions of "health" and "illness" are imposed. Until engaging with hegemonic norms of "health" and "illness," women with chronic illness remain without *specific* identities, and more easily link up with and de-link from nodal points around which *specific* identities may coalesce. Substantively, women with chronic illness scramble to find some sense of belonging to some community, but are disappointed when, because of their fluctuating symptoms of illness, access to various communities— women with disabilities, medical clinics, workplace environments, social circles—is denied by other people who have based their actions on specific interpretations of the constellation of symptoms the women have articulated to activists, physicians, employers, and friends.

RESITUATING OUR FOCUS

Instead of setting discourses of the body as the centerpiece of our analysis— those associated with medicine, health, illness, or disability—we chose to examine bodily experiences of women with chronic illness. The acknowledgment of this shift is important because it identifies our project as different from the ones we have discussed. We recognized that, from the conception of the project, we would work from women's experiences of body rather than from a theory of discourse. In making our way through feminist incarnations of psychoanalysis, feminist applications of Foucault's work on the body, and feminist elaborations of identity, we have been able to chart a path so as to conceive the relationship between illness and health for women with chronic illness as an "in between" identity. We read bodies as existing *through* corporeal sensations and meanings of body ascribed by discourses. Thus, instead of theorizing the "chronically ill body," we seek to understand the discursive body and the material body of women with chronic illness. In order to sort through ill bodies as both discursive and material entities, we think it best to contextualize women's experiences of chronic illness in their everyday lived spaces. We outline our approach to conceptualizing chronic illness and space in the following chapter.

3

❧

Conceptualizing Chronic Illness with Space

L ike works on theorizing the body, writings on space, too, have influenced our project. Having both been trained within the disciplinary boundaries of human geography, we have long-standing fascinations with space. We know that conceptualizations of space underlying theories of social phenomena, including the body, fundamentally affect the interpretation of information. Whether space is conceived as passive, relational, or constitutive influences understandings and explanations of those phenomena.[1] As our work has become increasingly interdisciplinary, we have found that space, though often accounted for, is not always integral to theory nor suitably conceptualized. This project provided us an opportunity to sort through what it means for us to spatialize identity and to account for the spatial aspects of the experiences of women with chronic illness.

Examining theories of bodies (see chapter 2) and space (see below) is not the only reason we undertook this study. For us, trying to understand chronic illness and the experience of women like Patience is just as important, and perhaps even the catalyst for our study. Bringing together theories of the body and conceptualizations of discourses about women with chronic illness entails exploring how bodily sensations of sickness and spatial contexts of ill bodies affect each other, expressions of identities, and experiences of being ill. This type of understanding goes beyond coming to terms with symptoms of fatigue, pain, and forgetfulness toward elaborating the context within which women with chronic illness live their daily lives. It is important to maintain our focus on *both* the manifestations of illness (as corporeal feelings) *and* the social, political, economic, and structural contexts of being ill for two primary reasons. First, to dismiss, disparage, or even devalue bodily sensations and feelings plays into the demeaning experiences of being ill that frame the lives of women with chronic illness. To excise the sensorial and emotional would undermine the integrity of women's experiences of being chronically ill. Second, how women with chronic illness live their lives is inextricably linked to their homes, workplaces, and social networks as well as their health care practitioners, insurance companies, and employers. To take a body out of its context would bolster idealized, insubstantial notions of what a body is and can be, ignoring the implications of what living *through* bodies looks like.

In the previous chapter, we focused on theories of the body and identity to show how conceptualizations of the body might affect our understanding of chronic illness. In this chapter, we turn to a discussion of *ill* bodies, as discursive and material entities. We use the metaphors of "in between" and "filtering" to position ill bodies spatially—literally and figuratively. We next discuss competing conceptualizations of space and offer a recasting of spatiality by highlighting constitutive notions of space alongside constitutive notions of body. We close by pulling together our ideas about bodies, chronic illness, and space as laid out in these two chapters.

ILL BODIES AS BOTH DISCURSIVE
AND MATERIAL

Situating our interests on ill bodies as discursive and material entities assists us conceptually in refusing the binary of discourse and materiality. We see the body as a nexus through which women with chronic illness experience both discourses and materialities of the ill body. Engaging with the literature on chronic illness has been a difficult task for us primarily because much of the work has been based on humanist values, something we have already rejected through our engagement with works theorizing the body and identity.[2] As well, some analysts in literature on chronic illness sometimes conceptualize chronic illness as "disruptive," not in the sense of resisting hegemonic relations of biomedicine or the like, but rather the putative normality of everyday life.[3] Often experience is conceptualized almost as an "essence," as something that takes place through *non-specific* bodies.[4] For us, "experience is an interpretation *and* is in need of interpretation."[5] Experiences of women with chronic illness are not in and of themselves tightly woven with fixed meanings; rather, they are open to contestation—not in the sense of denying existence but in the sense of providing contextual and deconstructive readings.[6] Making sense of women's experiences of chronic illness entails a close reading of both the meanings ascribed to particular experiences as well as the sensorial aspects of those experiences. These experiences, however, are not clearly differentiated between that which is discursive and that which is material. For example, we are only able to articulate pain by saying that we have pain. Even though the bodily sensation of pain exists in some manner, we make sense of it only through our articulation, our utterance, our communication. This articulation in words does not, however, move pain solely into the discursive realm, denying the material sensation of pain. Rather, after our articulation, pain remains a material sensation open to yet another discursive articulation, perhaps as somatic, sympathetic, or spiritual. This ontological conundrum is not our central interest; it serves merely to identify a particular point where discourse and materiality entwine to produce an understanding of an experience of a bodily sensation. Our focus is on the entwinement, to the point of simultaneity rather than unity, of the discursive body—through inscription, signification, complicity—and the material body—through activity, sensation, modification.[7]

Rather than risk reproducing modernist conceptions of wholeness as monolithic oneness, feminist critics have been careful not to set up casual oppositional binaries. Instead, the ground upon which feminists have problematized that which is part of neither side of the binary has been through the metaphor of "in between." The notion of being "in between" captures conceptually the areas linking the discursive body and the material body that have been to date left buried, unspoken, tacit. For feminist geographers, being "in between" is a popular way to describe the relational positioning of the feminist geographer to her research.[8] Being "in between" is also useful analytically when conceptualizing the processes through which multiple discourses constitutes self, identity, and experiences of the body.[9] Although being "in between" may evoke notions of distance (across which difference has been lain), we see that in these instances there is an implied sense of "being caught" between two things, not "fitting in," separate from, being somehow displaced and not as a distance to be traversed. How this (dis)-placement plays out through our experiences of body brings with it an unsettling disjuncture between the discursive body and the material body. Problematizing this connection is at the heart of our project.

Just as work on the body and identity influenced our conceptualization of the body, conceptual work on bodies "in between" affected our ideas about how we could make sense of women's experiences of chronic illness. The organization of literature on women's "in between" bodies, including works dealing with health and illness, reflects hegemonic notions of what a woman's body *should* be, outside what we conceive of as *specific* bodies.[10] Almost always, an ill body—whether discursive or material—is contrasted with the normative, healthy body, one free of disease, illness, or disability. Those works most influencing our thinking are those concerned with processes of meaning ascription, with concrete bodily activities in specific spaces, as well as those problematizing the relationship between discursive and material bodies.

One site where the dilemma of being caught between the discursive and the material is in mental illness. The experience of being mentally ill, no matter the cause, is disconcerting for the ones who are ill as well as those around them. Hester Parr makes this point in connection with how persons with mental illness navigate the spaces they live in.[11] She argues that disruptions in daily routines prompt persons with mental illness to devise and adopt various coping strategies, including taking drugs. In her research, she notes that youth living in the street tend to use non-prescription drugs whereas older people with longer-term housing tend to use prescription drugs. Regulating behavior through drugs produces what Parr calls the "medicated body." It should come as no surprise that she would find that people ensconced more tightly in the norms of society would want to conform more closely to hegemonic configurations of "acceptable" behavior whereas youth already resisting normative lifestyles would choose a coping strategy that would alleviate immediate symptoms rather than firmly control behavior not "acceptable" by prevalent norms of society. Our reading of Parr's medicated body, brings into focus the dissonance between the discursive and the material. Rather than only a resolution to alleviating symptoms or controlling behavior associated with various types of mental illness, we see the goal of medicating the body with drugs and other types of alternative drug therapies as an uneasy combination of both which can be recast as the realignment of the discursive body with the material one. In this sense, people with mental illness through medication are transformed from the irresolute "in between" into the comfort of "in the midst of."

The pressure to move from "in between" spaces into "in the midst of" poses its own sets of problems. Jennifer Terry recounts a history of the medical search for a biological base for homosexuality.[12] Because of the dominance of the discursive heterosexual body at the time of the emergence of medicine, any departure from that norm was deemed *deviant* and slated for clinical investigation. When, upon intensive scrutiny of the concrete, physical body, medical practitioners found no link between non-normative behavior and the body—either in "defective constitutions or degenerate genes"—they sited the deviance in the psyche.[13] These practices within nascent medicine fostered an environment that forces persons away from the indeterminable spaces of homosexuality and bisexuality toward spaces that could be accounted for, such as the psyche, and set into motion arguments that sexual deviance was a psychosexual desire by a small number of people. By the mid-twentieth century, the notion that only a small percentage of people engaged in homosexual behavior was shattered. Alfred Kinsey's work on sexual practices showed that nearly half of all men and a comparable number of women in the United States would in their lifetime engage in homosexual behavior.[14] Terry uses this historical shift in understanding the link between homosexuality and the body to argue that the homosexual body disappeared and was replaced by a sexualized body that was both heterosexual and homosexual, a boundary highly permeable and contingent. This replacement pushed the discursive homosexual body into a new space of "in between," one placed on a continuum between two "pure" types of sexuality. There is yet one more layer of Terry's argument that indicates the pressure to be "in the midst of" rather than "in between." Movement among gay rights activists to resuscitate arguments that homosexuality is biological sets up a political stance whereby homosexuals can claim to be the "way they are" because that is the way they are "hardwired."[15] Discursively, their advocacy opens up opportunities to argue that gay men and lesbians can be protected legally against discrimination and closes off claims that, through reform, homosexuals can once again be heterosexual.[16] This collective anxiety over who is "us" and who is "them" materially is part and parcel of pressuring persons into conformity through designating persons as "something" discursively in lieu of being outside normative categories. Yet, as Terry points out, there are indeed slippages between discursive and material positions—biologically, socially, and politically.

Slipping between assignations of a particular category over time has not been the pattern for women with "unexplained" chronic illness, at least culturally. In her comparative account of fictional representations of women's illness in mid-nineteenth century and at the turn of the twentieth century, Diane Herndl offers two ways of reading texts which prominently feature invalidism: as revolutionary texts resisting women's oppression and as hegemonic texts furthering the interests of the masculine power elite.[17] She argues that as cultural unrest, a theme across both periods, illness can be figured to represent political uneasiness and shift attention away from the "abstract, sociopolitical suffering of oppression to the concrete, bodily suffering in illness."[18] As a result, both women and failure are depicted as character failings, thus repudiating the material body. This repudiation also individualizes pain and illness, and reinforces the image of women as weak, frail, failing, and, subsequently invalid. This strikingly stable and rigid depiction of invalid women remained throughout the twentieth century to represent women with unexplainable debilitating physical symptoms, even though there was no constellation of symptoms promoting a similar phenomenon until the last two decades of the twentieth century. The increased frequency of the diagnosis of Chronic Fatigue Syndrome has many parallels with the illness of Neurasthenia, a popular diagnosis in the late 1800s and early 1900s. Susan Abbey and Paul Garfinkel give an account of these parallels and come to startling conclusions.[19] They argue that both illnesses emerged in a time preoccupied with "commerce and material success and by major changes in the role of women. Both have been labeled medical diseases and explained in terms of the major scientific themes of their day."[20] Rather than pursuing this line of argument and disentangling the processes through which women come to develop these particular physical symptoms in various cultural contexts, they prematurely halt their analysis and conclude that Chronic Fatigue Syndrome will meet the same fate as Neurasthenia, and become for the most part extinct at the turn of the twenty-first century.[21] They imply that there is a collective anxiety about the future and that women, in particular, perhaps because of their weak constitution, cannot physically muster strength and fortitude to face the unknown.[22]

Anxiety over becoming an "us" and designating a "them" collectively also plays out individually, increasing in intensity with respect to being cast as ill socially and culturally and to enduring the destabilization of the material body. Vivienne Anderson discusses how anxiety at the scale of the individual shapes everyday surroundings by drawing her experience with Scleroderma, or Progressive Systemic Sclerosis.[23] She recounts her struggle with physicians over the diagnosis, relates her daily life with her partner, and suggests ways to include these experiences in feminist theories of the body. For our project, we read her work as an expression of how the discursive and material bodies mutually constitute each other over time. Since the onset of her illness in 1980, Anderson has moved from being discursively incorrigible to discursively aligned having been assigned an accepted category of "chronic illness." Once "explained," a chronic illness becomes anchored in a particular material-based etiology. Concomitantly, competing explanations rooted in the psyche or psychosocial conditions fade, illness slowly becomes socially accepted,[24] and various treatment options are made available by health practitioners. This move is not permanent, "fixed" in time or space, or immune to further destabilizations. When new symptoms emerge, although she remains ill among her closest social contacts, physicians reclassify her ill status as "explained" to "unexplained," and consequently to "unbelievable." To be recast as "unexplained," Anderson, and women like her, once again experience the disjuncture between the alignment of the discursive and the material body. In comparison to Terry's analysis where there is slippage between categories over long periods of time as dominant discourses and social practices within medicine shift, in Anderson's work, the slippage is more immediate, taking place within smaller time frames and is concerned with discursive re-categorizations by persons with biomedical authority because of recent shifts in the material body.

But what if there is never an acceptable category to assign women with chronic illness? Women's experiences with chronic illness would differ dramatically if there were either a more constant category of disease of illness, such as diabetes, or a more unpredictable one, such as Multiple Sclerosis. This relative fixity shifts not only with biomedical authority but also with changes in social support networks. Being cast ill socially and culturally alongside bodily sensations of pain and fatigue together constitute the experience of the discursively and materially ill body. One evocative metaphor of their articulation is "filtering," or passing through one another. Heidi Nast and Steve Pile use this concept in the context of conceptualizing the link between bodies and places that invoke images of "keeping out, keeping back, defensiveness, interchanges, flows between, across, over, through places, through the body" as well as "cleansing, contaminating, fertilizing, washing bodies and places."[25] We like "filtering" because we can conceive the articulation of the discursive and the material as ones that pass through one another, sieving the other through its own existence. Neither dominates or subjugates; both are integral to each one's own expression. Many analyses that problematize the link between the discursive and the material body are not conceived as filtering, or as an expression of simultaneity. Rather, they are weighted toward one or the other, often with dire consequences for the concrete, physical, material body. Armando R. Favazza's work on self-mutilation and body modification bestrides psychiatry and cultural anthropology in attempting to bring the cultural and material body together.[26] He seeks to explain what is conventionally termed pathological behavior of self-inflicted pain and mutilation as well as belief-based rituals as means to gaining a sense of belonging, as fitting in, as part of a strategy to attain a "normal" life. He claims that scars from self-inflicted wounds, tattoos, intentional scarring, and other material remnants of body modification are reminders of interventions into the surface of everyday life. In terms of the discursive and material body, we read Favazza's work as an example of conceptualizing the body as primarily rooted in discourse that directs the boundaries within which a body can exist. Even though Favazza claims to embrace both cultural and physical aspects of the body, he remains within the realm of the discursive and concludes that self-mutilators are miserable with their lives and offers several types of therapies that are effective "cure." Fakir Musafar extends Favazza's work through what we would term "filtering" the discursive and material body by fusing the concrete act with the meaning ascribed to it.[27] Rather than pathologizing bodily activities associated with modification, Musafar suggests that "body play" is a way to attain a state of grace while still being fleshed, either by your own hand or by someone else's. Through his work as a body modifier, he shows that taking bodily modification seriously as both a process and outcome in a culturally sensitive manner enhances the experience of both the meaning of ritual and the awareness of sensorial ecstasy.

"Filtering" discursive bodies with material ones riddles each with the other to the point of simultaneity, where the meaning is indistinguishable from the concrete body. The inability to distinguish the two is not because they are the same,[28] but because they exist as a *specific* body at the same time. An effective way to loosen the relative fixity of the entwinement, disentangle the seemingly disparate elements of body, or sort through the complexities of the filtering process might begin with understanding the tension between women's sense of self and the relationship to the body. In her investigation of beauty and cosmetic surgery, Kathy Davis poses the relationship between the two as a dilemma, one that can embrace the ambivalence in a woman's sense of her own body.[29] Through her framework that draws out embodied subjectivity, agency, and morality, she gives a detailed account of the processes through which women undertake to alter their body permanently through cosmetic surgery. Going back and forth between what women think of their bodies and what choices they make and follow through in changing the physical appearance of their bodies, she is able to sift through discursive inscriptions of the drive toward an idealized body shape as well as specify the agency involved with women's decisions. Davis is quick to point out, in various ways, that the "sculpted body" in and of itself is not necessarily a non-feminist project through which women unwittingly comply with their own oppression. Rather, the sculpted body is a site to examine how reshaping the body is both desirable and problematic precisely because women can *both* recognize *and* be complicit with their own oppression.

These works that focus on bodily change are significant when talking about the bodies of women with chronic illness. Even though women with chronic illness do not usually self-mutilate (either because they are miserable or because they wish to reach a state of grace) or literally re-shape their bodies, they do engage in parallel sets of activities that meet the same ends. Women with chronic illness often turn to religion or spirituality to assist them in coping with the unknown fate of their bodies, especially if the illness is life-threatening as for example with Leukemia, Myelodysplasia Syndrome, and Scleroderma. The desire to deal with the impact of the disease process on the body—particularly in regards to pain—through attaining peace of mind stands in place of self-mutilation. As well, replacements for women whose joints have been ravaged by arthritis represent a way to sculpt the body—quite differently than the women who choose cosmetic surgery to re-make their body in order to attain the idyllic beautiful body. Nonetheless, the same realm of activity—surgery—is used to create a body whose functioning (albeit mechanical, and not discursive) is enhanced.

Holding in tension two apparent polarities is nearly unavoidable when thinking about chronic illness. There is always already an idealized healthy body lurking in the destabilized material body. Because the nature of illness is itself related to the concrete body, the filtering between the discursive and material is sometimes more easily recognizable than in other sites for investigating embodiment. Feminist analysts negotiating this tension have come up with widely divergent interpretations of the contexts within which illness takes place. Susan Bordo locates her examination of the body in the "many layers of cultural signification" that crystallize in the body as eating disorders.[30] Western culture is saturated with images of women's thin bodies—ones that have no fat, no bulges, no uncontrollable flesh—shaped through fitness, dieting, and surgery. Bordo argues that patriarchal values evident in consumer culture reinforce women's oppression by making women's "hunger as desire" a societal problem, thus creating the anorexic body. Women develop eating disorders because they attempt to embody these values where "self-determination, will, and moral fortitude" are replaced by actions that bring about a type of salvation, that is, "food refusal, weight loss, commitment to exercise, and the ability to tolerate bodily pain and exhaustion" lead to transcendence of the female body.[31] In contrast to Bordo's reading of cultural significations of the anorexic body, Abigail Bray and Claire Colebrook maintain that signification is "an active event rather than . . . the negation of some ground or the representation of some presence."[32] Instead of thinking about anorexia nervosa as an attempt to embody, or even to negate,[33] patriarchal values, they conceive "hunger as desire" which generates its own actions, ones that are not representative of some presumed essence or origin. When conceptualized as positive[34] activities, eating disorders become integral to self formation, not self destruction. Because anorexia is "a series of practices and comportments; there are no anorexics, only activities of dietetics, measuring, regulation, and calculation."[35] This intense numerical organization of the flesh continually generates more measuring activities. The discourses which then shape the body are those of regulation, control, and quantification and not slenderness, fitness, and patriarchy.

Both these analyses of anorexia nervosa filter the idealized body (the discursive) and the destabilized body (the material) through each other. Bordo privileges the discursive body by relying on signification as the primary form for interpreting the body. She understands body to be a site of inscription for culture. The body moves through discourses and takes on particular activities that would enable a woman to embody values inherent in the discourses she again passes through. While Bordo begins with discourse, Bray and Colebrook begin with concrete bodily activities. Through reading bodily activities as positive difference, they are able to loosen the "grip of culture" on the body and rearticulate concrete, physical activities with other discourses. They suggest that *as a body*, persons with anorexia might be better seen in connection with other bodies, signs, and social practices. They begin by refusing any single signifier for the body that would organize an interpretation of the body and are thus able to disrupt the foundational binary of discourse/materiality, and move more freely between the two. Thus, as Bray and Colebrook argue, conceiving anorexia as a set of practices of a specific dietetic regimen including, for example, counting calories, measuring food, and weighing, makes it easier to view anorexics as engaged in positive self production. This conception also makes it easier to trace these specific behaviors through discourses other than beauty, as for example linking the anorexic body to a "short-circuiting of contemporary practices of self-monitoring through quantification."[36]

In situating ill bodies for our project, we have used two metaphors, "in between" and "filtering," to draw out how ill bodies and those that are hegemonically and contextually defined as ill or sick are both discursive and material. In order to provide the beginnings of a framework through which we can understand women's experiences of chronic illness, we considered the work of diverse analysts who have either scrutinized the body as a site of being "in between" or problematized the connection between the discursive and the material as they play out on the body as nexus of inscription and activity. Holding in tension polarities inherent in our conceptualizations of bodies serves as the analytical departure point for our project, one that precludes privileging one pole over the other. As the works we reviewed in this section demonstrate, tension manifests more widely than just in thought's binaries. Indeed, they illustrate Foucault's point that all discourses and the social practices that sustain them have the potential to be dangerous. The series of acts that eventually deem *specific* bodies as deviant, such as those with bisexual desire, has similar features to those deeming other *specific* bodies as politically correct, such as those without surgical alterations. For our project, a dangerous move would be suturing the connections between the discursive and material too tightly, thus preventing new, innovative articulations of bodies to emerge. Pulling together the discursive and the material conceptually into unity, as a singular entity, would prevent the garish textures of bodies from entwining and manifesting in innumerable possible configurations. Conceptualizing the relationship between the discursive and material as simultaneous would actually promote dazzling assemblages of *specific* bodies. As a caution, with Foucault, we would note that through the constitution of each articulation of the body, there would not be anything making that specific body inherently liberating or oppressive. Yet being able to unravel the spatialities always already within the experience of ill bodies would assist in the task of exploring the body as a nexus of the experience of discourse and materiality and of disentangling how it is that bodies are constituted discursively and materially as *specific* bodies.

CONCEPTUALIZING SPACES

Efforts in medical geography to reconceptualize space in ways that permit a wider purview of social relations have benefited from studies in social geography. Graham Moon and Kelvyn Jones's call "to take space seriously" in the sub-discipline spawned discussion on the importance of including theorized notions of space in understanding all dimensions of health and health care.[37] John Eyles argued that within the discipline of geography, medical geographers in particular did not engage critical notions of space.[38] Interpretive space, conceived as human activities giving space meaning, and relational space, conceived as social relations creating space, were not widely used in medical geography even though they were regularly part of other sub-disciplines in geography, as for example, urban, economic, and feminist geography. Similarly, Robin Kearns and Alun Joseph made the case that if medical geography is to make a contribution to health research generally, then it is necessary to move beyond conceiving place as a nexus of ascribed meaning and space as geometrical dealing primarily with distance and proximity.[39] They suggest moving toward merging insights from socio-spatial and humanistic conceptions of space because

> [w]ithout considering the traditional power of space as an agent in the distancing or coalescing of resources, vectors, or people, studies of place are at best useful illuminations of the minutiae of daily life for people in particular places. And without an understanding of place to enliven the otherwise abstract and geometric spatial (b)landscape, our conclusions will be devoid of the human nuance and ambiguity that characterize the places in which we live out our lives.[40]

These types of works within medical geography paved the way for a shift in how health geographers understand the interconnections between health and place, space and illness.[41] The bottom line in these debates is that conventional notions of place as location and space as container need to be enriched by conceptions of space that integrate social relations from their very inception.

Relational and constitutive space have their origins in the notion of spatiality, a word used to connote several different meanings of the relationship between the social and the spatial since the rise of social relevance geography in the late 1960s. Throughout the 1980s, Marxist geographers elaborated the understanding of space as a social construction that actively reproduces itself.[42] By the late 1990s, spatiality had come to refer "not to a thing or object but to a process that produces the complex texture of capitalist social life."[43] With perpetual interaction, the social and the spatial continually construct and reconstruct one another, profoundly shaping everyday life. Edward Soja details the conceptual development of spatiality as a socio-spatial dialectic, a process in the context of explaining how capitalism can produce its own self-sustaining geographies.[44] He draws heavily on Henri Lefebvre's work on the social construction of space, whose notion that space is at the core of capitalist dynamics opened up materialist analyses of social relations.[45] Although separate, the social and spatial are ontologically intertwined, neither being able to break or merge completely with the other. It is up to researchers to sift through the constructed and contingent nature of spatialities. Critics claim that spatiality conceived as a socio-spatial dialectic, or even a trialectic when conceived with time,[46] cannot remain in the realm of Marxist geography and historical materialism because of the fluid ontological base Soja offers. Though never explicitly engaging or critiquing Soja's conceptualizations, analysts interested in space theoretically have continued to use the notion of spatiality. For example, Steve Pile, in collaboration with both Michael Keith and Nigel Thrift, also offers a tripartite vision of spatiality.[47] Rather than building on Marxist conceptions of the interrelationships between the social and the spatial, Pile begins with identity, the subject, and subjectivity. He draws on Jacques Lacan's differentiation of the Imaginary, Symbolic, and Real in psychoanalysis and then conceives spatiality as the links among images, signs, and that which is complete within itself. Together these spaces both constitute and are constituted by individual subjectivities. In stark contrast, Doreen Massey offers a different reading of spatiality, but comes to a similar conclusion regarding the constitutive nature of space itself.[48] Spatiality for her is more of a dimension of space recursively inclusive of social and economic relations coming together in space and time to produce and reproduce a particular place. She skillfully explores the entwinement of identity, subjectivity, and knowledge by linking the palpable, local spaces she inhabits daily with the systematic, global processes she and those around her are part of, resistant to, and complicit with. For Massey, the global and the local both constitute and are constitutive of individual and collective identity.

Common to these works using spatiality as a crucial concept in thinking about the social and the spatial is an implicit proposal to regard the project of theorizing space as both concrete and epistemological. There is no doubt of the need to understand how spaces we traverse in everyday surroundings shape who we are, our identities, and our subjectivities as well as how who we are and what we do shape spaces we inhabit. Our positionings within multiple sets of social relations matter, too, in conveying and constructing meaning of spaces and places. But this is not to say that these positionings determine either who we are or the meanings we ascribe to particular places; rather, they produce and create the social, the spatial, and the temporal indeterminably. Dilemmas arise when attempting to account for *specific* bodies through the concreteness of these interactions. Elizabeth Grosz identifies two prominent dilemmas arising when trying to understand the relationship between bodies and cities: cities either are a product of bodies or the body represents the city.[49] Grosz points out that, in an approach that conceives the city as a result of intentional acts of thinking humans, responsible for their origin, design, and function, the mind is privileged over the body and the relationship between the body and the city is clearly only one way. In an approach that conceives the body as analogous to the city and state, she draws attention to the gendered account of the body in the analogy, the perpetual binary of culture/nature, and the tendency to "naturalize" political relations as bodily functions. Underlying her refusal of both an external, causal relationship between the body and the city and a parallel, representational relationship, is a constitutive sense of space. She proposes instead viewing bodies and cities as "assemblages or collections of parts, capable of crossing the thresholds between substances to form linkages, machines, provisional and often temporary sub- or micro-groupings" wherein their relations involve "a fundamentally disunified series of systems, a series of disparate flows, energies, events, or entities, bringing together or drawing apart their more or less temporary alignments."[50] Through her discussion, Grosz offers an unfixed, non-determinist conception of spatiality, one where the inestimable number of potential constellations figure into the formation of the spatial. There are not multitudes of configurations vying for dominance; rather, there is a series of possible, fused, and fleeting intersections through which the social and the spatial emerge at any given time.

Using this transformed notion of spatiality we have drawn out of Grosz's work, we could argue that because of the constitutive nature of the relationship between bodies and spaces, *specific* concrete bodies always already have traces of the spaces they inhabit. We could also argue that the spaces we traverse also have indeterminable impressions of our bodies in their constitution. But do we want to make this argument? If we hold tightly to the claim that bodies and spaces constitute one another, how would we conceptualize a radical politics of the body? Would we need to be able to claim that we could intervene materially in these constitutive processes to direct and effect change? Or, would we need to spurn such claims and maneuver through our immediate, and perhaps our not so immediate, spaces and effect change *through* our constitution? Heidi Nast, to a certain extent, addresses the point we are making in her methodological piece about her cross-cultural work with women's spaces in Kano, Nigeria.[51] She re-tells three field stories where she negotiated social hierarchical differences among wives, concubines, and *bayi*,[52] not in a particularly ethnographic way with pen and paper, but "on the run," at the point of engagement. In one of the stories, she tells how she understood through her rudimentary Hausa language skills that a concubine called her an idiot. Nast turned to the concubine and asked, defensively, "*Who* did you say was an idiot?" The women responded with muffled murmurs. It was only later that she found out—through her patroness, the third royal wife—that she was wearing her headdress incorrectly and it appeared as if she were trying to pass herself off as married. Nast's story illustrates how her body contained traces of the spaces constitutive of her body and the spaces she then needed to maneuver through, yet the (visible) impression was ill-fitting, misleading; her material body in its substance and action created a glitch in the social fabric of women's spaces in the palace. Through this series of acts—unknowingly dressing improperly, being singled out for ridicule, responding defensively, feeling humiliated and shamed, realizing the source of the difficulty, writing the story—Nast documented in a fragmented way a micro-scale example of spatiality as a process by highlighting the notion that bodies and spaces change, not as a consequence of intentional intervention, but by acting (unconsciously) *through* constitutive processes. Had it not been for this particular configuration and manifestation of Nast's naïveté and her strong emotional response, neither the (momentary) rupture in the social fabric nor the constitutive reverberations would have ever taken place.

Although effective in illustrating our point about refusing claims that change takes place only through material intervention, unconscious or unintentional acts are not the only agents of change. Bodies and spaces are not locked into ceaseless, fixed patterns; they are only ever momentarily stabilized. The recursivity of constitutive relations, laced with power, permits the possibility of *deliberate* change. Another way to make this point is to extricate the argument from concrete bodies and think about theorizing space as an epistemological project. Epistemology concerns the realm of knowing and theories of knowledge. Space as metaphor has been integral to theories of knowledge in the context of power and identity.[53] Liz Bondi challenges geographers, feminists in particular, to rethink geographical metaphors in identity politics.[54] Taking on a spatial metaphor can be problematic because of the undertheorized notions of space and place that permeate Western thought. Unintentionally, space in an absolute, Cartesian, three-dimensional grid sense sustains metaphors like "place," "position," and "location" in discussion of identity, power, and knowledge. She advocates a spatially sensitive epistemology as a framework for understanding space as constructed and created in order to move beyond a fixed identity politics as a politics of *static* location. She reminds us, following Diana Fuss, that even constructivist approaches to identity have inherent in them an essence, a positioning, a subject-position.[55] Taking care not to reproduce simple, static notions of space is as important a task as taking care not to reproduce "inadequately conceptualized" notions of identity.[56]

Problems immediately arise when addressing the link between *specific* bodies and theorized space. If we can understand the link between concrete bodies and spaces as constitutive, how do we integrate bodies into epistemological space? Foucault's historical writings about power/knowledge are helpful in sorting through epistemological connections among bodies and space. Power, according to Foucault, is everywhere, operating through normalizing and naturalizing discourses and maintained by specific social practices and self-surveillance. In order to understand the entwinement and interdependence of power and knowledge outside the confines of the stringent notions of power to date, he uses the concept "power/knowledge" to address his central methods of inquiry—genealogy, archaeology, and ethics.[57] Power/knowledge provides analysis, historical and otherwise, with the ability to make intelligible particular configurations of social relations. Foucault argues that power/knowledge has been central in constituting bodily norms, any deviance from which regulates and disciplines concrete bodies through surveillance and self-scrutiny. Bodies, then, are discursively produced through disciplinary power which can be, and indeed is, resisted.[58]

Unfortunately, by Foucault's own admission, space is taken as an ontological given even though "geography necessarily lies at the heart of [his] concerns."[59] Making room for a spatially sensitive epistemology where space is conceived as constitutive entails more than considering "tactics and strategies of power";[60] it entails complexly integrating constitutive space into the notion of power/knowledge regimes. Spatiality as a process through which any possible, fused, and fleeting configuration of the social and the spatial emerges at any given time parallels Foucault's conceptualization of power/ knowledge, and when taken together creates power/knowledge/space. Inclusion of constitutive space in this way enriches explanations of disciplinary power and resistance of bodies. Without space, the very fabric of power/ knowledge becomes textureless, sensationless, dimensionless, producing disembodied accounts of the body.

MOVING TOWARD EMBODIED SPACES

This chapter has brought together some of our thoughts about the discursive and material body as well as the connections between bodies and space. A shared concern in these discussions of conceptualizations of body (depicted in the previous chapter) and space is the idea of constitution—discursive and material bodies are mutually constitutive, space is constitutive of the social and the spatial, and power/knowledge is constitutive of space. Bodies experiencing chronic illness provide an excellent opportunity for analysts to explore these ideas because women with chronic illness have experienced a destabilization of their bodies. Through interrogating this destabilization and subsequent negotiations of social and physical environments, we are able to identify disruptions in constitutive processes relating to discourse, materiality, identity, and spatiality. In that we do not accept mainstream knowledge as the basis for what we know, what we can know, and what is known, we can claim that what we present here, what we can derive from what we present here, and what knowledge there is in this presentation are partial; partial in the sense that we do not know everything and in the sense that anything that we do know or can know is incomplete.[61] However, even within this partiality, we can indicate how power/knowledge/space plays out in the lives of the women we talked with and how through their experiences we can speak of embodiment and embodied spaces. For us, embodiment refers to those *lived* spaces where bodies are constitutively located conceptually and corporeally, metaphorically and concretely, discursively and materially, being simultaneously part of bodily forms and their social constructions. Embodiment clearly is about inscription, the discourses being inscribed, and their corporeality. While living *in* and *through* space, bodies engage in material practices that produce and reproduce both the meanings of bodies, and the circumstances within which bodies exist. Through the notion of embodiment, we can begin to understand how Patience knows her body through the spaces she inhabits, how she undertakes to assess her bodily movements in light of bodily norms, and how she understands the disjuncture in her life between notions of illness and her experiences of chronic illness. Translating these ideas, notions, and conceptualizations into a framework for understanding experiences of chronic illness is the focus of the following chapter.

4

❧

Making Sense of
Chronic Illness

In order for a radical body politics to be able to have meaning for Patience
and other women like her in understanding experiences of chronic illness,
we need a way to make sense of the various aspects of bodies and spaces and
how they relate to discourse, materiality, identity, and spatiality. By "making
sense" of experience, we mean to offer an interpretation of chronic illness
that has already woven into it complexly textured conceptualizations that
challenge binaries prominent in thinking about bodies, particularly the
binary of discourse and materiality. Our intention is not to provide a definitive way to theorize body, conceive experience, or read ill bodies; rather, we
propose but one way to understand the experiences of women with chronic
illness, one rooted in our own re-thinking of bodily inscriptions and limits,
and in daily negotiations of subjectivity, identity, and space. Without relying
too heavily on the cultural significance of bodies or the play of words notable
in poststructuralist approaches to reading the body or premising our notions
on any essential category of bodily state of being or function, we seek to set
up a framework where reading bodies, particularly ill ones, as simultaneously
discursive and material is a matter of course. Through our engagement with
the theoretical works on body and space in the context of chronic illness we
discussed in chapters 2 and 3, we have produced visual representations that
serve as an assemblage of the concepts we think important in a radical body
politics. Delineating this particular constellation as a framework reveals our
approach to understanding the conceptual linkages among bodies and
spaces.

Central to our framework for interpreting women's experiences of chronic
illness are three sets of tensions organized around, first, "bodies in context";
second, corporeal space; and, third, embodiment. These tensions permit us

to situate our arguments vis-à-vis one another through critical conceptualizations of body, chronic illness, and space. This assists us in reaching our goal of a radical body politics that accounts for specific articulations of power and identity through women's experiences of chronic illness. In the rest of this chapter, we draw out in more detail a conceptual framework to help us make sense of *specific* bodies in *specific* environments. We describe the framework in three iterations. Initially, we present conceptual linkages visually and define concepts included in the three figures. In the second iteration, we describe more thoroughly the three sets of thematic tensions and show how they conceptually frame our interpretation of women's experiences of chronic illness. In the third iteration, we comment on a series of ideas that have influenced our thinking by showing how they relate to, but do not readily appear as part of, the framework. We close by previewing the empirical chapters that follow by noting their positioning within our framework.

A CONCEPTUAL FRAMEWORK

Iteration One

Figures 4.1, 4.2, and 4.3 are visual representations of the conceptual linkages we use to describe our notion of the body and its constitutive relations of identity and space. The first forms a conceptual building block. The second notes one way these building blocks might be put together. The third shows a more complex fitting. The two-dimensional representations (of three-dimensional objects) in figures 4.1 and 4.2 are somewhat limiting, but still convey the tenor and gist of our arguments. The three-dimensional representation is more difficult to read, but conveys more evocatively our ideas comprising the framework, even if in a truncated form. We intend that the following description fit all three figures, at the same time.

  Conceiving the body as a nexus through which women with chronic illness experience both discourses and materialities of an ill body shatters the notion of the body as a lone, separate, individual entity. Instead, the body is always already "in context," socially constructed and materially present, as part of a collective, imbued with power, and a political being. "*Bodies in context*" exist spatially in relation with other bodies, recursively constituted through tangible and intangible things and processes—escalators, street corners, apartment blocks, capital, income, race, knowledge, beliefs—at any given time and place. Being able to hold in tension the "body in context" with both the physical body and the processes that ascribe meaning to bodies, heightens our ability to understand identity as a never-ending process of becoming, in lieu of a static fixed label to take on or reject at will. Taking seriously this tension entails conceiving "bodies in context" as being embed-

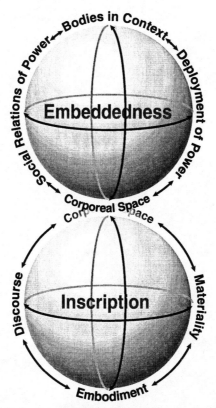

Figure 4.1. Basis for Conceptual Framework for a Radical Body Politics

ded within social relations of power, organized around ability, age, citizenship, class, ethnicity, gender, health status, nationality, race, sex, sexuality, and other sets of relations we have yet to name. This *embeddedness* expresses the relationships among "bodies in context" in specific arrangements of the deployment of power, as for example, colonization, domination, exploitation, marginalization, naturalization, normalization, oppression, and other hegemonic deployments of power we have yet to name.[1] Being embedded is always already in a state of tension because integral to embeddedness is the ongoing mediation and negotiation of the relations of power within a specific arrangement of a deployment of power. The intensity and direction of these mediations and negotiations are not predetermined for where there is power, there is room for both complicity and resistance—neither of which is ever fully intact, neither of which is fully refuted.

Experience of the embeddedness of "bodies in context" exists through *corporeal space*, an interim state within spatiality, constitutive of the discursive

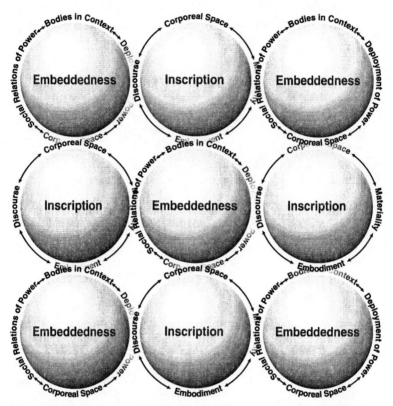

Figure 4.2. Linkages among Concepts in Conceptual Framework

and the material.[2] Corporeal space comprises the *living* spaces of "bodies in context," claiming both the temporal and spatial specificity of bodies, giving rise to *specific* bodies and *specific* environments. Corporeal spaces are tension-filled, coalescing around "bodies in context," filtering links between power and identity, encompassing that which is "in between," and shifting through reverberations of changing discourses (including language, text, and ideas) and materialities (in reference to both economy and matter, the latter inclusive of the physiological, biological, and anatomical aspects of bodies and the physical and substantial aspects of spaces). Holding in tension meaning and matter, corporeal spaces are able conceptually to maintain a synchronous union between the discursive and material so that bodies are neither wholly idealized, nor utterly fleshed—bodies and spaces are simultaneously idealized and fleshed, and are made *specific* through the recursive process of becoming.

Just as corporeal space is an interim state within spatiality,[3] so too is embodiment. For us, *embodiment* "refers to those *lived* spaces where bodies

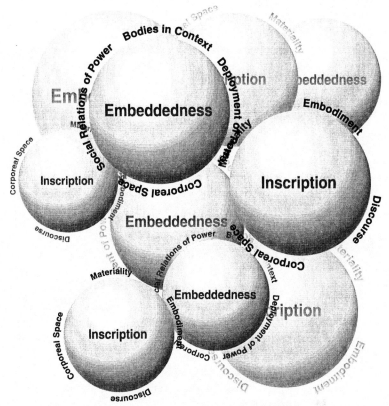

Figure 4.3. Three-dimensional Portrayal of Conceptual Framework

are located conceptually and corporeally, metaphorically and concretely, discursively and materially. . . . This means *being* simultaneously part of bodily forms and their social constructions."[4] Conceptually, then, embodiment holds in tension the specificity of a body and of a space, as a juncture point of the idealized and fleshed body, and the connection to other *specific* bodies through concrete practices—culturally, economically, politically, socially, and spatially. Through the process of inscription, bodies and spaces come to be constituted as *specific*. We conceive *inscription* as a set of concrete processes, including both discursive and material practices, that etch onto a body a particular rendering of an idealized or fleshed body. They are coded and are made culturally intelligible through readings of the embodiment of bodies in context. These inscriptions are not only surface markings made available for public and private scrutiny; they are integrated into subjectivity and identity through recursive constitutive processes.[5]

Iteration Two

These three sets of tensions—"bodies in context," corporeal space, and embodiment—in combination with embeddedness as a state of being and inscription as a process, deal with similar aspects of body and space while differing in their focus and intensity. "Bodies in context" focuses on the placement of *specific* bodies in relation to each other through recursive constitutive processes—socially and spatially. Through "bodies in context," for example, collective identities emerge which form the basis for political action through a cooperative politics. As well, because "bodies in context" are in a state of becoming, politics are not predictably stable; as power shifts or is deployed through a different configuration of social relations, *specific* bodies de-link and re-link with other "bodies in context" and form yet another configuration. The mediation of the tension already implicated in embeddedness is what creates the path for various linkages, de-linkages, and relinkages to take place. What comes to matter in a radical body politics is the apparent solidification of this embeddedness or a "fixing" of a particular set of linkages that can then produce strife.

For example, conflict may arise in a workplace situation when a woman with chronic illness negotiates a reduced workload at the same pay rate as her coworkers. Workload and pay rates are ensconced in and an integral part of any working environment. When apparent "fixities" like these are contravened, "bodies in context" may clash, that is, when a woman with chronic illness de-links from what is expected in terms of workload and re-links to a differently configured set of tasks at the same pay rate, then her coworkers may become disgruntled because it would appear that the woman with chronic illness is receiving preferential treatment. In our illustration, embeddedness is merely an ontological expression of the relationships among "bodies in context" and specific arrangements of the deployment of power and is neither essentially "good," "bad," or "indifferent." Negotiating tensions around "bodies in context" within specific arrangements of deployments of power permits a radical politics to emerge so that women with chronic illnesses can restructure their environments to accommodate the disease process.

Corporeal space and embodiment, too, are concerned with the relationships among bodies and space. Corporeal space brings into focus the articulation (and manifestation) of the embodiment of "bodies in context" while being embedded in a particular arrangement of social relations. This is not a matter of scale, where scale is the manifestation of size in a nested hierarchy of space.[6] Rather, corporeal space exists at multiple scales wherein each envelops "bodies in context" that exist discursively and materially. Corporeal space is also where *specific* bodies negotiate inscription and experiences of physical and social spaces and begin to make sense of their embodiment, their lived spaces where the experience of meaning and matter are fused, inseparable, happening at the same time. Shifts in embodiment can spark changes in corporeal space, as for a simple example, pain in the lower back and shoulders while sitting at a desk ignites a transformation of the desk into an ergonomic workstation. Or, a shift in discourse can inscribe bodies as deviant in one place but not in another, as for example, being openly gay in a small town in the U.S. Midwest may be inscribed as deviant whereas in New York, it may not. But embodiment is not always so isolated, singular, or episodic. Embodiment is integral to the expression of "bodies in context" and is in itself imbued with power and situated within specific arrangements of the deployment of power.

In reading figure 4.1, the links among the sets of tensions are outlined clearly, with the exception of the link between embodiment and "bodies in context." A clearer representation might appear in the form in figure 4.2 where a tapestry of links unfolds. Yet the most evocative array of linkages among the three sets of tensions appears in figure 4.3 where spaces of embeddedness and inscription intersect and overlap with power and its deployment, discourse, and materiality. Still, none of these images captures our argument entirely. Some questions we address—what constitutes "bodies in context," corporeal space, and embodiment? Through what processes do collective identities emerge? What constitutive relationships exist between the social and the spatial? Whereas others we elide, how are gender and sex related? How are specific arrangements of the deployment of power related to *specific* bodies? What is beyond the sphere of body politics? Though problematic, we still find these figures and their description useful in assisting us in our elaboration of a radical body politics in that they (a) outline the conceptual path we have taken to our interpretation of women's experiences of chronic illness, (b) provide definitions of concepts we consider significant theoretically, and (c) lay the groundwork for expanding our understanding through our empirical work in the following chapters.

Iteration Three

But before moving on to our interpretations of women's experiences of chronic illness, we find it useful to discuss in more detail topics that have been part of working out the intricacies of the framework that may not necessarily readily appear as part of our figures. These topics—experience, embodiment, analysis, spatiality—have all been integral to our thinking about body politics, our interpretations of women's accounts of living with chronic illness, and to the formulation of the project itself.[7] We go into more detail about embodiment because our thoughts as written so far do not capture the richness of the concept to convey the complexities of everyday life. The following discussion is a series of comments that we do not attempt to pull together until the end of the chapter. We suggest holding in tension the framework as presented above, including the figures, with what we present in the following few sections. Also important in reading our attempt both to fill in the lacunae emerging in our thinking and to challenge our rendition of theory is to remember that we are not setting up a theory to apply to a set of data; rather, we created this framework out of our own immersion in the women's accounts of chronic illness.

Experience

Unlike Joan Scott's suggestion that it might be better to do away with "experience" so as not to commit the crime of essentialism in an intellectual environment that ever-increasingly shuns such ideas, our choice is to "trouble" experience in a way that challenges the notion through scrutinizing the context within which acts constituting the experience take place.[8] Teresa Ebert's arguments about the limits of knowledge in feminist theory are somewhat useful in thinking about radical body politics in that she indicates what feminists should concern themselves with when dealing with theory.[9] For Ebert, experience is an already mediated understanding of an act that cannot be separated from the understanding and explanation of other social practices. Part of her argument relies on contrasting how two notions of "critique" conceptualize limits to knowledge. On the one hand is immanent critique "which reads the text or system in its own terms and sets its limits or blind spots—its aporia—as the result of the contradictions or self-division.within the text of system itself."[10] She points to deconstruction as a useful method in siting these aporia. On the other hand is historical materialism "which begins with immanent critique but refuses to confine its inquiry to the internal contradictions and differences of the text or system."[11] These internal contradictions are always linked to larger social contradictions relating to race, gender, and class. Ebert then goes on to argue that the limits to knowledge in feminist theory are not only located within feminist theory, but also, as an historical entity, are the "effects of the operation of the social relations of production as relayed through the dominant ideology and power relations that constrain and restrict what it is possible for us to see and know."[12] Some feminists' unease with engaging in critique is rooted in conflicts over the notion of what theory is. Ebert refers to those satisfied with immanent critique as antitheory theorists, who claim that any theory is totalizing and universal. In contrast, she wants us to understand theory as an explanation of historical intelligibility, which can lead more easily and effectively to a transformative politics. At the center of Ebert's recasting of theory is experience— either in the humanist notion of a moral self (cultural feminism and writings from women of color) or in the postmodern notion of the ethical subject of pleasure (ludic feminism and *jouissance*). What is at issue about experience in her arguments are *the circumstances within and through which a series of acts constitute themselves as an experience.*

Ebert's critique of feminism assists us in thinking through, first, the notion of what a limit is and, second, figuring out what it is we want out of theorizing experiences of ill bodies. If we are to be consistent with Ebert's claim of experience being already mediated and her line of reasoning about feminist theory needing to move beyond immanent critique, then we must think through how the discursive and material limits to ill bodies articulate with "bodies in context" and attempt to contextualize individual experiences of ill bodies with social practices. For women with chronic illness, limits of chronically ill bodies are mutable—confining one day and liberating the next. This inconsistency brings into focus the indeterminableness of bodies with chronic illness as either ill or healthy, either abled or disabled, either marked with a culturally intelligible diagnosis or unmarked visibly with bodily symptoms that can, at least for a while, be denied publicly. "Bodies in context" are *specific* bodies in relation to one another, their bodily activities already mediated, ones recursively constituted socially and spatially. Being able to theorize the relationship between bodies, their limits, and context, or what we call their embeddedness, can keep concrete bodies with chronic illness intact through their abstraction, without having to break the connections of experience and its context.

In "troubling" experience, we also found autobiographical writings useful as a way to understand the fluctuating limits of the discursively ill body and the materially ill body.[13] Feminists have shown that engaging autobiography analytically can provide insight into phenomena hitherto neglected, denied, or simply unseen.[14] Numerous autobiographical accounts in the chronic illness literature exist, mostly rooted in phenomenology, and rarely in feminist, poststructuralism, or critical theory.[15] One exception is Margrit Shildrick and Janet Price's work with chronic illness.[16] Shildrick and Price question their "own differential responses and those of others to the constitution of Myalgic Encephalomyelitis (ME)—which is the diagnostic category assigned to one of us [Price]—as an unproblematized nexus of experience."[17] Price's illness was the catalyst for their re-thinking of disabled bodies. By drawing on Price's experiences of support groups, they argue that in having as a goal a medical definition of ME, ME support groups are naturalizing the experience of ME into a collection of symptoms that can and should be readily identifiable *as ME*. Once recognized as a disabling disease, then people suffering from ME can be categorized as *disabled*. Shildrick and Price point out that these activities reproduce the disabled body as unknowing victims of disease, perpetuating the normative identity of disabled bodies as helpless bodies needing support from charitable citizens. Their use of autobiography analytically supports their claim that postmodern feminists need to deconstruct the processes of normalization and naturalization that designate an

identity of being disabled and to lay bare the ways the body itself is constructed as being stable and fixed as disabled. These feminist autobiographical writings have pushed our thinking about experiences of chronic illness,
particularly in the areas of experience and embodiment. We found that the
only way we could differentiate analytically the context of the *experience* of
chronic illness (that is, *the circumstances within and through which a series of
acts constitute themselves as an experience*) from the corporeal spaces of women
with chronic illness was through conceptualizing the relationship between
the two as one of inscription—material and non-material etchings of discourses about chronic illness onto destabilized and destabilizing bodies.

Embodiment

Through our attempts at "troubling" experience through feminist autobiographical writings, we were better able to grasp what embodiment actually
meant for us. In the feminist literature on the body, definitions of embodiment are abundant, for example, through holistic conceptions of approaches
to life, an ethical stance in the provision of care, and a way of gaining knowledge of the world.[18] Even with all this choice, we were left with an uneasy
feeling that embodiment was something different than what we were reading
about. We tend to gravitate toward works that conceived embodiment about
being, about ontological assumptions, about existence—whether referring to
individuals or groups of individuals. For example, David Harvey and Felicity
Callard both emphasize Marx's notion of the sensual body and seek to re-
establish a body-based materiality to our understanding of the embodied
nature of the labor process.[19] Harvey argues that the body is at once a site of
political-economic contestation and of the very forces that construct it.
Bodily practices that can arise out of engaged labor, which sometimes create
unhealthy bodies contradicting capital's need for healthy bodies, and the cir-
culation of variable capital, are a means to transform relations of production
and create an emancipatory politics. Callard bases her argument on this type
of Marxist production-oriented analysis with subtle infusions of poststructural thought. Situating her arguments at the intersection of Marxist and
queer theory, she suggests rethinking the connections between the laboring
body and the corporeal configurations that give rise to particular meanings
of the body. She pushes Harvey's arguments further and shows that there are
lessons to be learned from looking at the "body" historically, especially how
bodies were integral to the emergence of industrial capitalism.

    These conceptions of embodiment focus on the contexts within which
bodies exist and act. In thinking about chronic illness, experience, and autobiography in the context of bodily and knowledge limits, we tried to understand embodiment as a place where bodies "fit" into society and as an
account of our corporeal existence. We found intriguing definitions espoused

by Seyla Benhabib and Elizabeth Grosz. Benhabib defines embodiment as "the self develop[ing] an *embodied* identity, a certain mode of being in one's body and of living that body" . . . "through the social-historical, symbolic constitution, and interpretation of the anatomical differences of the sexes."[20] In this definition, embodiment describes a state of being, one that maneuvers through discursive inscriptions as a living entity. What seems to be missing in this casting of embodiment is the connection to the fleshed body as something other than fundamentally given. Grosz links embodiment directly to the corporeal body and argues that

> bodies themselves in their materialities, are never self-present, given things, immediate, certain self-evidences because embodiment, corporeality, insists on alterity, both that alterity they carry within themselves (the heart of the psyche lies in the body; the body's principles of functioning are psychological and culture) and that alterity that gives them their own concreteness and specificity (the alterities constituting race, sex, sexualities, ethnic and cultural specificities). Alterity is the very possibility and process of embodiment: it conditions but is also a product of the pliability or plasticity of bodies which makes them other than themselves, other than their "nature," their functions and identities.[21]

Through alterity, Grosz makes explicit that concrete, specific bodies emerge as something other than themselves through discourse and materiality. Alterity permits a process of embodiment to take place as both the means and the medium through which *specific* bodies become *specific* identities. This connection between bodies and identities, although useful in understanding identity as something other than an ascribed social construction, remains perpetually suspended in a spatial void because it lacks what Benhabib made central in her conceptualization—an ontological notion of embodiment as bodies being lived.

One of the difficulties addressed in these works, as well as others,[22] is attempting to break free of the ontological neatness of having a pre-discursive body. Abigail Bray and Claire Colebrook, for example, think through embodiment in terms of the re-linking body image and its consumption.[23] They draw on Deleuze to claim that "ethics is the way in which bodies become, intersect and affirm their existence,"[24] which is indeed another definition of embodiment. In trying to break free of the pre-discursive body, they focus their attempt on sorting through the process of the imposition of representation or how representation orders its meanings. They argue that thought, discourse, and reason are indeed bodily events, producing their notion of embodiment.[25] In concrete terms, this means that diseases like anorexia nervosa are *bodily activities* rather than the presumed notion of the material manifestation of the *negation of the body*. For other chronic illness, this might manifest as: illness and inscriptions of illness are bodily activities and not deviant in comparison to a "normal" body—either materially or discursively. These activities have "real" consequences for what one can and cannot do. Illness can be seen as not being *un*healthy, but as merely being— without having to be compared to a "standard," a "normal," or an "ideal- ized" body.

Because we seek to be sensitive to the ontological simultaneity of discourse and materiality, we want to refuse both pre-discursive and pre-mattered bod- ies.[26] Thus, attention to the ontological status of the body when conceiving embodiment is important. In conceptualizing embodiment as the contexts within which bodies exist, we build on the strength of Bray and Colebrook's insight that discourses are bodily events and not materializations of thoughts and ideas. The discursive involves ideas, notions, thoughts, images, and texts of/about the body and the material includes sensuality, biology, and physio- logical processes. But embodiment is more than just being about the *juncture* point of a discursive and material entity; it is also about being connected— temporally and historically—to other discursive and material entities—other bodies—in concrete practices, politically, culturally, socially, and economi- cally. We want to re-think bodily activities, bodily forms, and bodily imagin- ings as embodied, in ways that refuse to break connections among the elements within processes that constitute bodies as textured entities.

Analysis

No matter the framework, when any study, narrative, or analysis is pre- sented, readers—both lay and academic—assess the study's plausibility, "validity," and "accuracy" in various ways. Questions arise: "Does this make sense?" "Does this make sense in light of other studies on the same topic?" "Does this make sense given what I know about related topics?" Resonance with one's own experience is often forefront in assessing the accuracy of the analysis. We are no exception for we tend to "accept" analyses that fit within our own worldviews. We make this point with regard to being able to read analyses of embodiment critically. We have been astonished at just how seductive analyses can be. By *seductive* we mean the commonsense-like man- ner in which some analyses are presented such that it makes it difficult for a listener, reader, or critic to disagree with, make objections to, or challenge the interpretation. A tight, well-organized, well-thought out presentation of research or theory produces what can be referred to conventionally as a rigor- ous, high-quality analysis. It would "make sense." It would resonate with experience. It would "fit" the existing worldview. And, if the analysis is par- ticularly good, to disagree might even appear as a moral transgression.

At the same time, the same analysis can be narrowly restrictive, closing off interpretation or interactive discussion that could be useful in figuring out or imagining different ways to think embodiment, bodily activities, and "bodies in context." We may be seduced into thinking that this particular analysis is indeed *the* way to think about embodiment because it makes so much sense. Different ways of thinking embodiment are closed off because we cannot engage with the presentation of the material that supports the analysis. We may accept it as a type of "truth." One analysis that we found particularly seductive is Alexandra Howson's piece on individual women's narratives about Pap smears as a specific cancer-screening behavior.[27] Most of the women whom Howson talked with agreed that routine Pap smears were a *commonsense* thing that women just do—"get used to it," "an every-day thing," "something which just had to be done," and "something that women should go and get done."[28] She interpreted their stories in the context of governmentality and argues that the women's stories exemplify what Bryan Turner terms a "Foucault paradox."

> In contemporary capitalist societies, citizenship may be underpinned by welfare systems which provide a greater degree of equality of opportunity in relation to healthcare. Where health is increasingly perceived as a desirable, though limited resource, the state is also required to provide a correspondingly greater degree of control over its populations. In this respect, citizenship is broadly considered as a series of individual rights and entitlements, therefore, the paradox is that *the provision of citizenship, of which health is an aspect, entails greater surveillance and social regulation by quasi-governmental organisations and agencies.*[29]

This initiation of and active control over surveillance is what is at issue for Howson—also known as a regulated body.

In order to place Howson's analysis into a context that we can use for elaborating our framework, we need to review briefly two pieces of Michel Foucault's work. Insight into discipline of the body was the focus of Foucault's work in *Discipline and Punish* and *The Birth of a Clinic.*[30] According to Foucault, discipline produces "docile bodies" that are subjugated: "Discipline increases the forces of the body (in economic terms of utility) and diminishes these same forces (in political terms of obedience)."[31] Through this subjugation, bodies are disciplined by external scrutiny and self-surveillance. Intense external scrutiny coupled with normalizing pressures serve as ideal surveillance mechanisms for society. Foucault demonstrates in his history of the prison that with the introduction of the architectural structure of the Panopticon, an observation tower in the center courtyard of an annular building, punishment was transformed into a disciplinary mechanism through a constant visual supervision. Yet it is important to note that Foucault argues that emergence of the prison was not "laws, codes and the judicial apparatus" but rather was the effect of numerous carceral mechanisms fuelled by the power of normalization.[32] The deployment of power/knowl-

edge, as Foucault repeatedly points out, is involved in a multiplicity of disciplinary networks—including for example medicine, psychology, and
education—that support new disciplines which are "becoming ever more
rigourous in their application."[33] He maintains that the problem now "lies
with the steep rise with the use of the mechanisms of normalization and the
wide-ranging powers, through the proliferation of new disciplines, they
bring with them."[34]

Similarly, in *The Birth of the Clinic*, Foucault demonstrates that through
shifts in the discourse of medicine, particularly at the time of the French
Revolution, the body became a site to map and disease became no longer a
collection of symptoms, but a series of malfunctioning organs, tissues, and
chemicals. With the aim of making the hidden parts of the body more obvi-
ously perceptible, "new" medical doctors sought a space to visually modulate
the functioning of the body as well as to poke, prod, and vivisect them. More
than just a place for investigation, the clinic needed a system of orderly activities so as to produce a unified account of the body. Particular organizing
conditions necessary for the emergence of the clinic were those of a systematic understanding of the body, a separation of medical expertise and ill bodies, and a homogenous space for the patient—culminating together in the
power of the clinical gaze.[35] Just as with the discussion of the discipline of
the body in *Discipline and Punish*, Foucault repeatedly points out that medicine is but one of the more "visible witnesses"[36] to the restructuring of the
way in which experience is constituted. Having the body, as a nexus of experience, the object of a scientific, medical gaze changes the structuring of subjectivity.[37]

In Howson's analysis, she claims that there is slippage between Foucault's
notion of regulatory and disciplinary power and that of his use of the Panopticon. She claims that the shift from surveillance to self-surveillance is
wrapped up in the centralized power notion implicit in the Panopticon. As
a result, the multiple resistances to the deployment of power/knowledge are
not a focus of inquiry because analysts in sociology tend to concentrate on
"*practices* of surveillance instead of *experiences* of self-surveillance."[38] Casting
cervical screening as a surveillance technique sets up Howson's analysis of
the experiences of women either getting or not getting smears. Through her
interpretation, Howson sees that compliance to cervical screening is shaped
by the discourse around being a "good citizen." She systematically shows
that the women actively engage and seek out this preventative measure. She
also shows that the social networks they belong to are influential in determining whether or not they get smears—a family member receives an abnormal smear which sets off a reaction where several other family members get
smears. She argues that this is one way the women negotiate the surveillance
of their health and take control of their health care. She uses the concept of
embodiment to translate the women's experiences. She defines embodiment
as "the dialectical process between embodied experience and the language

available to articulate such experience. Hence, the notion of embodiment refers to a process of transformation and mediation in which embodied experience is authentic and articulated through cultural categories."[39] She comes to the notion of *embodied obligation* to describe the active participation in health surveillance. She links the practice of getting a smear to being a good citizen by interpreting the ways in which the women describe the experience of getting a smear through the discourse of good citizenship.

We see that there are two seductions going on here—one is in the women's stories themselves and the other is in Howson's analysis of the women's stories. First, with regard to the women's stories (as presented by Howson), why would someone not get a smear regularly? Most women know about it, and know that it is useful in detecting pre-cancer and cancer cells. They describe it as a regularized, routinized, commonsense behavior for all women once they become either sexually active or begin menstruating. The seduction here *is* the normalization of cervical screening—constructing cervical screening as common sense, refuses its construction as a state-sponsored monitoring of potentially diseased citizens. In precluding this second reading, the possibility of being both common sense *and* state-sponsored monitoring is also precluded.

The second seduction—that of Howson's analysis—obscures this reading of the process of normalization as part of health self-surveillance. What happens is that the analysis itself is seductive—she sets her argument up for thinking about citizenship, and doesn't permit other readings of the women's stories. The concept of *embodied obligation* makes sense given her analysis, which is plausible, valid, and rigorous. But its use precludes inclusion of other discourses that shape the women's articulation of their experiences, as for example, health, fear of dying, fear of being ill, fear of violation, sexuality, femininity, or motherhood.[40] Because she talked only to women who did get smears and analyzed their articulations of bodily experiences, she unintentionally creates another dichotomy and sets up women who do not get smears regularly as being "bad citizens." Even though Howson's purpose was to provide an example of how women negotiate their sense of embodiment, she sets up the notion that embodied experience and its articulation is linked only to one discourse. What is not clear is how that one particular discourse is chosen as part of either resistance or self-surveillance—is it rooted in theoretical readings? In the words of the women themselves? In philosophical questions? In the women's senses of embodiment? Because she presents her analysis so well (so seductively), her analysis closes off other possibilities, as for example, linking cervical screening to other discourses such as fear of developing cancer, privacy, body image, or health promotion. The story becomes one of being "good," and, inadvertently, not being "bad," and not only of just citizenship but also of personhood, binaries that also need undoing.

Spatiality

Foucault's work in *Discipline and Punish* and in *The Birth of a Clinic* assists us in understanding how normalizing mechanisms in the case of the women with chronic illness discipline the body. Disciplinary networks made up of physicians, alternative health practitioners, employees, employers, coworkers, family members, insurance agents, and claims adjusters constitute the ways in which the bodies of women with chronic illness exist within and beyond their limits while at the same time engaging them. What is significant in the women's accounts of living with chronic illness are the ways in which they engage their physical and social environments through the processes that constitute these spaces as environments as places wherein women with chronic illness can or cannot be ill, that is, their spatialities.

Spatiality is the array of processes that articulate with one another to produce the complex textures of social life. It is not the simple outcome of spatial contexts, such as being ill in the home or visiting the doctor's office. Rather, spatiality involves the processes constituting the home as a place of literal and symbolic refuge and the doctor's office, a place of healing. The idyllic meanings a culture ascribes to specific places shape the choice and desire to be in certain places while ill, as for example, at home or the doctor's office, and not at the mall or traveling. The material aspects of physical spaces permit individuals to "recover" from being ill—including things like privacy, familial or paid assistance, prescriptions, and professional health advice. Together discursive and material processes constitute specific spaces as "appropriate" and "inappropriate" places to be ill.

Spatiality is not easy to demonstrate empirically. Specificities are not only difficult to pin down, but often seem trite when discussed, as for example, having access to your own private bathroom. But these sorts of qualities that plausibly characterize spatiality, indeed spatialities, do not preclude a spatiality from being depicted, experienced, explored. "Space . . . forever illuminates and creates the social as it absorbs and propels its texture, character and fabric."[41] The social and the spatial are inextricably linked forever present within the other. One way to get at spatiality is to situate experience, subjectivity, and identity in that web of social relations and processes of power and bring to bear the inscriptions of textured "bodies in context."

USING THE FRAMEWORK

The conceptual framework we outlined in this chapter is our assigned starting point for our interpretation of women's experiences of chronic illness even though this is not where we began. The tensions among "bodies in context," corporeal space, and embodiment that make up the substance of our approach to understanding women's experiences of chronic illness, emanated from our readings of the women's accounts of living with chronic illness. For us it became clear that discursive and material bodily inscriptions are integral to sorting through how women negotiate their corporeal spaces and form identities individually and collectively. In a discussion about being ill, being healthy, identity, and identity politics, it is important for us to conceive the body as both real and figurative, both material and discursive, both sensual and textual. Materially, our bodies circumscribe our existences. In this sense we are sensual beings, ones that are tactile, emotional, and sensorial. With chronic illness, women feel pain, fatigue, disorientation, fear, malaise, frustration, alienation, isolation, anxiety, and excitement. At the same time, our bodies carry cultural markers that tag us as aged, raced, sexed, classed, sexualized, disabled, and ill. Because of the complex ways individuals and groups of individuals are embedded in various social relations of power, and constitute and are constituted through these same relations, particular practices of power (congealing in a specific arrangement of the deployment of power) creates a wide variation of identities. It makes sense to claim that women can be both complicit in their regulation as women with chronic illness and resistant to normalization processes of biomedicine, their bodies both a·site of oppression and a site of resistance. The corporeal spaces, where women live, think, act, and feel, recursively constitute "bodies in context" through multiple discourses and various aspects of materiality. Bodies can be both ill and healthy, both abled and disabled, and be neither ill nor healthy, abled nor disabled. Refusing categorization is an option. Because of the openness to fluctuation and change conceptually, constitutive social and spatial process produce the body as a complex nexus comprising contradictory, competing, and paradoxical inscriptions. Yet we must remember and incorporate into our understanding that individual women experience these inscriptions simultaneously as a fusion of both meaning and matter, space and context. And, it is in this sense that we can say women embody chronic illness.

We drew out this framework from the theoretical work we discussed in the previous chapter and from the women's stories of their daily lives. Thus far, we have only discussed theories, concepts, and notions of bodies and chronic illness, an important albeit incomplete elaboration of a radical body politics. Our approach has been deeply influenced by our engagement with the stories the women with chronic illness told. In order to provide a fuller depiction of our approach to understanding women with chronic illness, we need to demonstrate our arguments and flesh out our framework by drawing on the experiences of *specific* bodies. In each of the four empirical chapters (chapters 6, 7, 8, and 9), we interpret women's experiences of chronic illness in light of four themes: the discursive, the material, identity, and spatiality. This thematic distinction is merely a way to organize our interpretation, for all are part of the ontology of the experience of chronic illness. Yet in order to make our way through the fleeting, fluctuating, and unstable corporeal spaces of women with chronic illness, we need some way to "trouble" experience. Through these chapters, it becomes clear that we make sense of women's experiences through interrogating the embodiment of women, their corporeal spaces, and their expressions as "bodies in context."

5

❧

Approaching Analysis and the "Interpretive Act"

The conceptual framework we have presented is informed both by insights from the theoretical literature we have discussed and by women's accounts of living with chronic illness. While our theoretical discussion, in part, precedes the women's "voices," it is grounded in their narratives of their everyday lives. The following chapters draw directly on in-depth interviews with women diagnosed with either Myalgic Encephalomyelitis (ME) or Rheumatoid Arthritis (RA). Data from the interviews are used to further elaborate and substantiate the ideas outlined in our conceptual framework. In working through the empirical chapters, it becomes clearer that we work with theory and empirical material together, moving between each as each informs the other. In this chapter, we begin with a brief discussion of working with theory in the research, and how we have used interview data from this study in the context of presenting our discussion of the women's accounts of their everyday lives. We go on to place ourselves in the research, considering how working together, but from quite different positions, has informed the analysis. Next we describe the design of the study, including recruitment, methods, and the process of the research. We conclude with information about the women who took part in the study to provide context for the quotes and passages drawn on in the following chapters.

CONSIDERING SOME METHODOLOGICAL ISSUES

Using theory in research requires a delicate balance between "letting the data speak" and analyzing data with the aid of sensitizing concepts from theory.

In what is now something of a classic, Clifford Geertz spoke of the outcome of this process in terms of "displaying the logic of their ways of putting them [things] in the locution of ours."[1] Since the time Geertz wrote, researchers using qualitative research methodologies, particularly in feminist research, have recast the terms of producing knowledge in emphasizing the importance of "their" words being part of a bottom-up, collaborative process in reaching "ours," meaning the analytic concepts of representation.

Following the crisis of representation during the mid-1980s in ethnography, there has been considerable discussion of "reflexivity," or the exercise of reflecting upon the myriad ways location of the researcher in a research process conditions the knowledge that is constructed. Feminist researchers have perhaps been the most vigilant in pursuing the implications of recognizing the "interpretive act" as the core of research—determining, not just shaping, what comes to be presented as some sort of truth claim. While the social location of the researcher vis-à-vis that of study participants has attracted most attention, other dimensions of "positionality," such as geographical location or the various and unstable points of connection and disconnection between researcher and study participant have been considered less often.[2] In this chapter, we do not claim to make our positioning in this research project completely transparent, nor could we; what we do is contribute to the discourse of how feminists use qualitative methodologies.[3] We are aware of the complex dynamics of interviewing and the ways that layers of context at different scales will have influenced what we asked and what we were told in the specific sites of the interviewing.[4] But our purpose is not to interrogate the interview process. Rather, we focus on our location—as part of both reflexivity and as coming to the analysis, or "the interpretive act"—from different spaces.

WORKING WITH THEORY AND DATA

The in-depth interviews produced many pages of transcripts on which the analysis of the following chapters is based.[5] Inevitably, we "see" data through preconditioned lenses, which focus not so much on what we see as how we see it, although the two are not mutually exclusive. For example, codes may be assigned to specific phrases, paragraphs, or sentences with some degree of consensus in that such a phrase, paragraph, or sentence can be bounded in some way. The conceptualization of that "bibbet,"[6] "scrap," or somewhat longer passage from the transcript will, however, be informed by what the analyst brings with her in terms of her life experience, grounded in structured relations of power, and theoretical knowledge. This "fact" surrounding qualitative analysis is well rehearsed, although its meaning is tempered by work that considers all knowledge as situated and partial. Reflexivity that intends to make transparent such life experience and theoretical positioning is likely to lead to disappointment, for it is nigh impossible to examine completely the situatedness of knowledge.[7]

Even so, we still think it important to consider our own locations as we work through our analysis. In the next section, we engage in some conversation about how the analysis involved both synergies and tensions as we worked in developing concepts from and in conjunction with data. Before moving toward indicating our locations, however, we point to a way of working with data that is not a disjuncture from the inductive methods commonly discussed in the context of ethnography, but more consciously an occasion to work *with* data in order to *elaborate* theory. This involves first steps of coding data and identifying descriptive or substantive and conceptual themes emerging from data. Then, from this first cut at analysis, we draw particularly well-articulated commentary, or "mini-case studies," for illustration and support of the theoretical ideas being developed. Thus, rather than relentless descriptions of every woman's account of pain, malaise, belief, disability application, structural changes to the home, struggles with her employer, and the like, we use a forcefully expressed account of a particular event that captures what it is we are trying to convey. We do not want to invoke discussions of typicality, archetypes, or representativeness—all of which presume a clear distinction between theory and data. Rather than clustering a number of quotes from women to illustrate themes emerging from the data in an empiricist or descriptive fashion, we have selected quotes for their particular aptness or manner of articulation that helps us develop our theoretical argument. It is to be emphasized that these are not unusual in terms of any other woman's way of describing her experience and concerns; indeed we select quotes, passages, or mini-case studies that capture emotions, concerns, or experiences that were usually discussed or talked about in some manner during the interview.

Our choice of focusing on particular women's narratives, however, helps to provide some texture to the women's "voices," especially the longer quotes and passages that provide some context for a single or a set of issues brought up at that point in an interview. The tables in this chapter further assist in contextualizing our selections for they provide demographic information which indicates something of the women's structural position and recent work history (see tables 5.1 and 5.2). Although the study involved both women with ME and women with RA, their accounts are not used evenly; rather they are used as they aptly articulate a point of discussion. While there were some commonalities in experience, the nature of ME and RA as chronic illnesses differ substantially in some respects as can be drawn out from discussion in the following chapters.

Table 5.1. Socio-economic data including source of income for women diagnosed with ME

Pseudonym	Age	City	Education	Individual Yearly Income[a]
Agnes	71	CRD	Trade School, BSW, MSW	$26,500
Alex	44	GVRD	College	$21,500
Brie	57	GVRD	BA	$8,220
Caron	51	CRD	BA, MSW	$26,400
Connie	60	CRD	Trade School	$19,920
Debby	37	GVRD	BA, BSW	None
Dolores	44	CRD	College Degree in Nursing	$24,000
Elise	44	CRD	BSW, MSW	$60,000
Erin	38	CRD	Grade 12	$8,220
Gina	47	GVRD	MSW	$6,200
Janice	33	GVRD	BA	$14,400
Jayne	53	CRD	BEd	$37,680
Julia	40	GVRD	Trade School	$40,000
Leeza	54	GVRD	Business College	None
Pauline	55	GVRD	BA	$25,000
Raquel	54	CRD	College Degree in Interior Design	$33,600
Reann	33	CRD	BSc, MSc	$22,560
Sandra	late 30s	CRD	College Degree in Dental Hygiene	$14,950
Shelagh	43	GVRD	College	None
Sophie	61	CRD	Trade School	$36,780
Stella	57	GVRD	High School	$24,000
Teresa	49	CRD	Trade School	$8,220
Verna	late 40s	CRD	BA	Not reported
Vivienne	40	CRD	BA	Fluctuating
Yvonne	33	GVRD[h]	BA	Not reported

Notes:
[a] Incomes were self-reported. There may be discrepancies in amounts reported.
[b] In order to maintain confidentiality, some income sources were not reported, such as trusts, real estate, and support payments.
[c] "Own" implies there is a mortgage. We note the status of the mortgage only in the cases where the mortgage is paid off. Additional fees are also noted.
[d] Description of household members are self-reported. We use the terms the woman used. "Partner" does not indicate sexuality.

Table 5.1. **(continued)**

Pseudonym	Source of Income[b]	Profession or Employment	Tenure[c]	Household Members[d]
Agnes	State Disability Pension, Old Age Pension	Retired	own; no mortgage	self; husband
Alex	State Disability Pension, Long-Term Disability Insurance	Banking	own	self
Brie	State Disability Pension	Psychological Testing	rent	self
Caron	Long-Term Disability Insurance	Social Worker	own	self; husband
Connie	Long-Term Disability Insurance	Secretary	own	self; husband; two teenagers
Debby	Mother	Student	n/a	self; mother
Dolores	Long-Term Disability Insurance	Nurse	own	self
Elise	Employed as Counselor	Counselor	own	self; partner
Erin	Social Assistance	Retail	own; no mortgage; maintenance fees	self
Gina	State Disability Pension, Life Insurance Disability Benefits	Social Worker	own	self; husband; three teenagers
Janice	Employed as Teacher	Teacher	own	self; husband; two teenagers
Jayne	State Disability Pension, Long-Term Disability Insurance	Teacher	own; no mortgage	self
Julia	Employed in several retail positions	Retail	rent	self
Leeza	Husband	Homemaker	own	self; husband
Pauline	Long-Term Disability Insurance	Social Worker	own	self
Raquel	Long-Term Disability Insurance	Project Manager	own	self
Reann	State Disability Pension, Long-Term Disability Insurance	Technician	own	self; husband
Sandra	Employed as Healthcare Provider	Healthcare Provider	own	self; husband; two school-aged kids
Shelagh	Note: State Disability Pension denied	Homemaker	own	self; husband
Sophie	Long-Term Disability Insurance[e]	Technologist	own	self
Stella	Ex-husband	Homemaker	own	self
Teresa	Social Assistance[f]	Nurse's Aide	own; no mortgage	self
Verna	Employed as Community Organizer	Community Organizer	own	self
Vivienne	Student Research Contract Work	Banking/ Student[g]	own	self; partner
Yvonne	Father	Student	rent	self

[e] Sophie appealed the long-term decision to cut off her benefits in 1998. She succeeded.
[f] At the time of the interview, Teresa's state disability claim was under review. Her application has since been granted, increasing her income to about $12,000 per year.
[g] Vivienne was in banking at the onset of ME, but was a student at the time of the interview.
[h] Yvonne found out about the study in the GVRD, but at the time of the interview she lived in the Fraser Valley.

Table 5.2. Socio-economic data including source of income for women diagnosed with RA

Pseudonym	Age	City	Education	Individual Yearly Income[a]
Alice	58	CRD	Trade School	$30,000
Angel	76	GVRD	High School	$18,000
Barbara	34	GVRD	High School	None
Belle	28	CRD	BEd	$10,800
Bette	60	GVRD	Grade 12	$12,000
Carolyn	45	CRD	BA	$9,000
Charlotte	50	CRD	College Degree, Administration; Some university	$19,200
Eve	43	GVRD	BED	$30,000
Fern	56	CRD	BA	No Disclosure
Gwen	70	GVRD	Grade 9	$10,200
Helen	45	CRD	Some college	$12,000
Inge	49	GVRD	College Degree, Nursing	$20,000
Janet	36	GVRD	Some university	$36,000
Jeannette	36	CRD	BA; Some graduate work	$21,000
Lila	42	CRD	College Degree, Nursing; Some university	No disclosure
Margie	40	GVRD	Some college	$10,000
Mary Ann	31	CRD	BA	$24,000
Nicola	36	CRD	College Degree, Secretarial Work; Some university	$21,600
Noreen	42	GVRD	BA	$15,400
Renee	42	CRD	Some college	$8,500
Rhonda	34	GVRD	BA, MA	$35,000
Ronnie	36	CRD	BA	$8,400
Ruth	41	GVRD	College Degree, Electronics	$9,700
Sara	73	GVRD	Grade 12	$10,800

Notes:
[a] Incomes were self-reported. There may be discrepancies in amounts reported.
[b] In order to maintain confidentiality, some income sources were not reported, such as trusts, real estate, and support payments.
[c] "Own" implies there is a mortgage. We note the status of the mortgage only in the cases where the mortgage is paid off. Additional fees are also noted.
[d] Description of household members are self-reported. We use the terms the woman used. "Partner" does not indicate sexuality.

Table 5.2.   (continued)

Pseudonym	Source of Income[b]	Profession or Employment	Tenure[c]	Household Members[d]
Alice	Private; State Disability Pension	Retired	own; no mortgage	self; husband
Angel	Old Age Pension; State Disability Insurance	Retired	rent	self
Barbara	Husband	Flight Attendant	own	self; husband; three school-aged kids; nanny
Belle	Employed as Tutor; Provincial Disability Grant	Tutor	n/a, parents own	self; mother; father
Bette	Long-term Disability Insurance	Office Worker	rent	self
Carolyn	State Disability Pension; Provincial Disability Grant	Counselor	rent	self; 24-hour attendant
Charlotte	State Disability Pension; Long-term Disability Insurance	Social Worker	own; pad rental	self
Eve	Employed as Teacher	Teacher	own	self; husband; three teenagers
Fern	Husband[e]	Homemaker	own	self; husband
Gwen	Old Age Pension; State Disability Insurance	Retired	own	self
Helen	State Disability Pension	Counselor	rent	self; husband; two school-aged kids
Inge	Employed as Nurse	Nurse	own	self; husband; two teenagers
Janet	Self-employed Consultant[f]	Consultant	rent	self; husband; boarder
Jeannette	Long-term Disability Insurance	Student	own	self; two teenagers
Lila	State Disability Pension	Student	own	self; husband
Margie	Receptionist	Receptionist	rent; subsidy	self
Mary Ann	Long-term Disability Insurance[g]	Office Worker	own	self; two roommates
Nicola	Long-term Disability Insurance[h]	Civil Servant	own	self; husband
Noreen	Employed as Counselor	Counselor	rent	self; roommate; three school-aged kids
Renee	State Disability Pension	Banking	own	self
Rhonda	Self-employed Consultant[i]	Consultant	rent	self; husband
Ronnie	Partial State Disability Pension[j]; Provincial Income Supplement	Contract Manager	rent; coop	self
Ruth	State Disability Pension; Provincial Income Supplement	Manager	rent	self; one teenager; roommate
Sara	Old Age Pension; State Disability Insurance	Retired	rent	self

[e] Fern refuses to apply for the state disability pension because she does not "feel" justifiably "disabled" to claim a benefit even though she cannot be employed because of RA.

[f] Self-employment for Janet emerged after a breakdown of the company where she was employed. This arrangement was not part of an accommodation strategy.

[g] Mary Ann changed careers and is now in sales.

[h] Nicola must apply for the state disability pension after having two years of long-term disability support. This is a common clause in long-term disability insurance benefits policies.

[i] Self-employment for Rhonda emerged as an accommodation strategy with her employer.

[j] State disability pension is linked to employment. Provincial grants are not. Ronnie is not eligible for a full state disability pension because she was not in the labor force long enough.

OURSELVES AND INTERPRETATION

As authors and interpreters we are located differently in this research. Here we signal where this became important to the analysis. Pamela's original interest was understanding the paid and unpaid work of women with chronic illness. However, after the writing of the proposal for this research, Pamela became ill and was diagnosed with ME. Her research trajectory changed drastically, moving away from questions about the labor process toward issues of destabilizing bodies and fluctuating identities. She was able to merge her interests in senior women constituting their home environments with the destabilizing bodies of younger women who were active in shaping their home and work environments on account of chronic illness.[8] Her own struggles over legitimating competing inscriptions of illness too fed her interests in other women's experiences of chronic illness, especially ME.[9] The overt politicization of her own positioning in her workplace while ill provided fodder for her ongoing political activism on campus and in the community.[10]

In contrast, Isabel's relationship to the research is not from a position of autobiography, at least not on the dimensions of chronic illness or disability. She shared common threads with some of the women, such as experiences of motherhood, postsecondary education, and class positioning, but not the experiences of living with a diagnosis of chronic disease, a destabilized body and identity, and the struggles associated with these that we recount here. Her interest in the research and the ground from which she was looking at the data was closely related to an earlier study on the experiences of women with employment after diagnosis with Multiple Sclerosis (MS).[11]

Data from Isabel's study and a study of Pamela's formed the basis of a discussion of conceptualizing the links between environment, chronic illness, and women's bodies that has also informed the study and discussion of this book (as we have already noted in chapter 1).[12] We note the "in between-ness" of women with MS and women with RA. There are parallels and differences with both, depending on the severity of the symptoms of MS for particular women, the course of the disease process (which is variable), and its visibility or invisibility for particular women. Like the women of this study, many issues revolved around medical and personal uncertainties, destabilized bodies and identities, and re-learning bodies and spaces. Such parallels and distinguishing features with some women with MS and some women with RA, and other women with RA and women with ME have been invaluable in sorting through the significance of what is different and what is similar for women with chronic illness who have different disease processes, different diagnoses, but share material and discursive destabilizations.

While we share similar research interests, although positioned within them differently, our location in other respects differs. Pamela is in a state of transition. At the beginning of the project, she was ensconced in a geography department teaching social planning, regional development, and cultural geography. Now she is part of a graduate program in policy and practice where she teaches applications of theory in social and health services and research methods in changing institutional contexts. A central purpose of the courses she teaches in the program is to challenge students to effect political change in "the system" through their graduate research and professional practice. Gaining insight through autobiographical writing is one analytical method she finds useful in teaching how to develop a critical practice—one where the practitioner (for example, a social worker, nurse, recreation worker, community activist, counselor, or child and youth care worker) is sensitive to her clients' and her own embeddedness as well as their and her own complicity with and resistance to dominant power relations. Pamela also uses the "results" from the research as a way to enact a community politics around issues concerning the practicalities of everyday life for persons with ME, as for example, accessing biomedical knowledge and knowledge about developing particular treatment regimes. She regularly meets with individual women recently diagnosed with ME to provide support and has given numerous talks about the volatility of ill bodies. Although she does not necessarily recount women's experiences of illness, she does present and discuss the theoretical ideas she has drawn from the women's accounts of chronic illness.

Isabel's interest in *using* the research relates to her location in academia, teaching students who intend to become health professionals, namely occupational therapists. Such students are typically embedded in a science paradigm and are educated under the umbrella of the health sciences that are broadly located within a biomedical frame of reference. At the same time, core principles of their intended profession emphasize the importance of the environment in shaping people's everyday occupations and responses to illness and disability. From her research, Isabel brings insights from health and social geography to understanding the broad concept of environment and fosters the further development of a social, rather than medical, model of disability within the parameters of occupational therapy theory and practice. This is a very different type of "political action" than that of Pamela, instead challenging the tendency in health science of a taken-for-granted acceptance of biomedical discourse, by showing it to be a cultural discourse grounded in and supported by an established power/knowledge nexus. Noting its power of definition and categorization and that it is not a homogenous discourse allows students to think through the implications of resistance to the cognitive authority of biomedicine for themselves and their clients. In addition, exposing the relations of power that condition the lives of women with chronic illness and promote disabling conditions helps to reveal that "context" is not just an individual matter of personal support systems and hostile physical environments. She is able to explore with students the complex relationships among health, disability, gender, race, and place, for example.[13]

In working together, we therefore bring experiences from different personal and professional locations to how we have approached the research and the interpretation of the women's accounts. The outcome of the synergy and tensions of our ongoing discussion is reflected in the analysis presented here—constitutive of the tensions of working through concepts that may represent the experiences of one of us but not the other. In the next section, we describe the study methods, recruitment process, and how the research process itself played out.

THE STUDY—METHODS AND PROCESS

We conducted in-depth interviews with 49 women living in Victoria (Capital Regional District, CRD) or Vancouver (Greater Vancouver Regional District, GVRD), British Columbia, who had been diagnosed with ME or RA.[14] For those women with ME, in the CRD, we contacted eleven of the women through the sole ME support group on southern Vancouver Island and three women through other community networks. In the GVRD, we contacted three women through a local ME support group and eight women through local "snowballing" with initial recruitment through a local women's center. For those women with RA, in the CRD, we contacted seven women through two local support groups and an additional three women through contacts we made from these groups. Two women were recruited through other community networks. In the GVRD, we contacted seven women through local arthritis support groups, three from the same women's center we used to recruit women with ME, and two additional women through "snowballing." All but one of the interviews were taped and transcribed verbatim by six different transcriptionists.[15]

During the interviews, we gathered information about how women with chronic illness structure their physical and social environments through discussions about the diagnosis, labor in the home and the workplace, and social expectations of being a woman. When designing the project we thought it would be useful to think about the discursive aspects of the diagnosis together with the material conditions of the illness. What we didn't expect was that, in the on average hour and a half long interviews, the women would consistently spend half the time talking about the diagnostic process. Because of the way in which we contacted the women for the study, we had recruited only those women who had already been diagnosed with either ME or RA.[16]

We chose ME and RA for a number of interrelated reasons. We knew a bit about each illness. ME, popularly known as Chronic Fatigue Syndrome (or CFS)[17] is a disease of the central nervous system with no known origin. Primary symptoms include fatigue, pain and muscle weakness, immune dysfunction, and cognitive impairment. For diagnosis, a person must have debilitating fatigue, sore throat, swollen glands, and low-grade fever for at least six months.[18] Other symptoms include sleep disturbance, overwhelming fatigue lasting for days after minimal exertion, migratory pain, sensitivity to light touch, migraine-like headaches, forgetfulness, imbalance, light-headedness, foggy thinking, vertigo, clumsiness, multiple infections, noise- and photo-sensitivity, nightmares, irritable bowel syndrome, blurred vision, anxiety, weight fluctuations (either weight gains or weight losses), and nausea. Rheumatoid Arthritis is an autoimmune disease, a type of degenerative arthritis, primarily affecting the joints. Unlike osteoarthritis, RA is systemic, affecting multiple joints at the same time. Major symptoms include hot, discolored, swollen joints, pain, and fatigue. Other symptoms presented include fuzzy thinking and forgetfulness. Diagnosis is through blood tests—a positive RH factor or a sedimentation rate of erythrocytes in a vertical column of anticoagulated blood under the influence of gravity for one hour.[19]

Similarities in the manifestation of the symptoms made the two illnesses comparable. Both affect predominantly women and both, initially at least, have symptoms that are "invisible." Maneuvering through this invisibility frames the employment choices women with chronic illness have. The highly variable nature of the symptomatology of both forces the woman into situations where flexibility is crucial, both physically and emotionally, to the progression of the illness. Given that neither illness has a cure, adaptation and adjustment socially and physically must presumably be ongoing. Differences between the two illnesses made us think that this might be a useful combination to explore ways to adjust to everyday life accommodating chronic illness. With ME, there does not seem to be permanent organ or tissue damage, unlike RA which ravages the joint and fuses bones together. In intense episodes of ME, symptoms largely remain invisible whereas with RA intense episodes leave marks on the body where the disease has transformed joints, reshaping fingers, knees, hips, and feet, impeding mobility and dexterity. ME is a contestable illness, one that was only designated by the Centers for Disease Control (CDC) in Atlanta, Georgia, as a disease in 1994. Even more recently, a group of Canadian physicians set diagnostic criteria for ME in 2001. RA is a more accepted illness in society, largely through the results of foundations like the Arthritis Society heightening public awareness.[20] ME has no conventional treatment regime except to reduce stress, rest, and do minimal exercise. RA has a range of standard treatments ranging from multiple types of therapies, such as physio-, hydro-, and massage therapies, to a host of drugs including analgesics, non-steroidal anti-inflammatory drugs (NSAIDS), glucocorticoids, and disease-modifying antirheumatic drugs (DMARDS).

In addition to these rather straightforward reasons, there were other motives underlying our choice to look at ME and RA. At the time of conceiving the project, Pamela had been involved with another project with seniors living with arthritis.[21] The purpose of that project had been to sort through the various ways seniors adapted their immediate environments to accommodate the disease process, especially with regard to assistive devices, physical adjustments, and home and office renovations. She found that the study, because of the way she designed it, had no way of accounting for the fluctuations in the seniors' everyday lives. The accounts of daily living she solicited from the women (and men) appeared static because of the focus in the interview on the changes already made to their environments and not the process through which they came to make those changes. Isabel was in the midst of a project that explored the everyday lives of women with Multiple Sclerosis. She focused on both the home and working environments of these women. She found that most of the women found ways to negotiate their spaces with their fluctuating symptoms. With this changeability of the physicality of their bodies, their identities, too, underwent change. When combining these interests, we decided to look further in depth in the lives of women with RA, especially those in the workforce. This would complement both studies. We also thought that we might get a better sense of the fluctuation Pamela missed in the arthritis study and Isabel identified in the MS study if we were to talk with women who suffered from a relatively less well known and relatively more unstable non-progressive disease process. We also both knew people who were diagnosed with ME, and had been struggling with symptoms for a number of years.

Once the interviews were transcribed, we "mapped" the narrative showing in detail what the women talked about. The interview guide was not overly structured and the content, aside from the general topics we outlined earlier, was directed by the woman with chronic illness. These mappings were useful in that they told us what sorts of topics women tended to focus on and what ones they tended to quickly address. Pamela then coded the transcripts according to details—symptoms, medications, vitamins, health supplements, treatments, friends, family members, encounters with physicians, jobs, descriptions of the workplace, money, attitudes toward health-related phenomena, emotions, descriptions of self, health, well-being, coping strategies, changes to physical environment, renovations, assistive devices, leisure activities, and exercises. A sorting and sifting of data at that point brought on another round of coding along the lines of diagnosis, employment, power, finances, biomedicine, spirituality, and social networks, followed by a third round indicating themes constituting discourse, materiality, identity, and spatiality. Between each coding session, we continued to read and engage with feminist theory on body, illness, and space. As we became further immersed in the transcriptions, the more intrigued we would become with a particular topic. We would then investigate new theories from different analysts in order to delve deeper into the topics we came across. Through our reading, we were able to "pick up" on the different meanings of illness the women were conveying as well as the material circumstances giving rise to particular actions by the women. This type of interaction, or "interpretive act," between readable accounts of experiences and explanations of their constituent parts enhanced our readings of the transcripts *and* the theory, enriched our analysis, and provided the substance for our radical body politics.[22]

THE WOMEN

We compiled socio-economic profiles of the women that are presented in tables 5.1 and 5.2, the former for women with ME, the latter, with RA. Information included in these two tables does not describe the women in their entirety. These descriptors only indicate social and economic status and are not intended to define status or define the women. All the women were white, ranging in age from 28 to 73. Four women self-identified as lesbian, with the rest identifying as heterosexual.[23] We want to make clear that these women are not representative of women in Victoria, Vancouver, or B.C., nor are they representative of women with ME or RA. Instead, the accounts these women provided us are illustrative of the everyday lives of women living with chronic illness. These data then, as presented here, merely set up a milieu within which to "place" in context these women and their accounts. In the following chapters, we make use of their stories in the form of quotes, passages, and mini-case studies to demonstrate a point we make about a particular topic. We draw on the women's accounts unevenly, not because some experiences are more valid than another. Rather, we do so because one woman's words might be more concise, more extensive, or more to the point.

In presenting our analysis, the support for our radical body politics, we organized our thoughts into four chapters. We want to emphasize that *all* these chapters are about living with chronic illness day to day. None of the accounts included in the chapters is separated from the everyday living spaces of women with chronic illness. We patterned the analysis in this way so as to heighten the principal aspects of our arguments. In chapter 6, through the women's stories of onset of illness, we concentrate on the discursive constructions of illness by examining the process of the destabilization of the material body and the search for a diagnosis. In chapter 7, we focus on the materiality of bodies, illnesses, and spaces by scrutinizing the women's accounts of limits they have encountered because of their illness. In chapter 8, we turn to poring over the constitution of subjectivity and identity in light of the stories the women told of their notions of their "self." In chapter 9, we look at the spatiality of daily lives of women living with chronic illness.

6

❦

Destabilization of the Material Body: Onset, Diagnosis, Inscription

I guess I was lucky not having to fight with Danielle this morning. Now that she's off to work, I can get ready for class. . . . More construction. I'll have to go the back way. . . . I'm not depressed. It helped at the beginning to know that there was something wrong with me. But not now. I'm not depressed. . . . Pay attention. . . . What if I had my life back the way it used to be? Well, maybe not with Ross. But my body. What if it were like it used to be? I could be working full-time, cycling to work, kayaking on the weekends, having the energy to parent Danielle. In the way that I want to and the way that she needs it. . . . I can't do any of that. Maybe, if this "thing" ever goes away, I'll be able do all those things again. I could have an herb garden just out the back door, and. . . . If it weren't for that day in November, when my neck started hurting. It really hasn't been the same since then. I thought I had pulled a muscle cleaning the bathtub. Who would have thought that all these years later, I'd still have the same pain. Not me, that's for sure. . . . No one knows I'm sick. Well, I guess there are some people that know. Okay, maybe quite a few. . . . But I don't want them to pity me. I don't need their help. I don't want them to think of me as "sick" or, ooh, what if they thought of me as ill? . . . Gee, I could be that person cycling to work. . . . What if I didn't have a car? What if I didn't drive? I couldn't bear to stay at home all day, every day. What if I get worse? Am I going to have to quit? . . . Stop thinking like that. Start thinking about class.

Onset of chronic illness destabilizes the material body making it unsteady, unsettled, unreliable. Depending on the disease process, speed of onset, types of symptoms, and body parts involved vary. Illness might take hold over the course of an evening, beginning with nagging pain in the ankle. Or illness might develop more slowly, taking years to pinpoint a source for a sense of malaise and migratory pain throughout the body. Once the disease process begins, manifested by a momentarily fixed collection of particular symptoms, the materiality of the body shifts unpredictably and changes the relationship between what the body can do and be and the expectations of what the body can do and be.

Initially, this destabilization seemingly affects only the material body. At onset, health appears to deteriorate while illness gains ground. Symptoms intensify, bodily sensations fade into one another. Alongside losses in muscular control, perhaps there is short-term memory loss. Physicians and medical specialists initiate an investigation of this deterioration by taking case histories, running diagnostic tests, searching for a cause, ruling out some illnesses, and uncovering possibilities. Because this destabilization of the material body is not a straightforward process, adjusting to onset of a chronic illness emotionally and psychologically can be distressing, upsetting, and disconcerting. Symptoms fluctuate from month to month, day to day, hour to hour, and can even roam from body part to body part over short time intervals. Such instability can prevent women from being able to communicate how they feel to family, friends, and health care practitioners and to figure out which specific symptoms seem to cause the most difficulty. While following the unexpected fluctuations of bodily symptoms, women are also forced to deal with the destabilization of the *notion* of a healthy body. A healthy body is often a taken-for-granted state of existence, particularly among younger women. Continuing sickness is usually associated with the elderly and the dying. Outside age-specific notions, chronic illness is often linked to coming from a "bad lot," having "bad luck," or being involved in "bad living." The former two rouse feelings of sympathy, compassion, and pity, whereas the latter provokes scorn, reproach, and blame. Dealing with this burst of emotions is disorienting and exhausting, often contradicting nascent feelings of acceptance emerging from within. Maneuvering through this process of destabilization, women exist in a state of ceaseless instability poring over symptoms of illness and meanings of health hoping to restore a sense of coherence.

In their quest to "put their body back together again," women persist in searching for a reason for feeling poorly by seeking out a diagnosis and associated treatments to "cure" the illness. Through diagnosis, women's ill bodies are made culturally intelligible. Diagnosis, central to biomedicine, legitimates an ill body by *naming* a specific disease process and so permits access to particular modes of treatment. Delivery of health care services in North America is organized primarily around disease categories that are determined through investigation based on scientific method and applied by holders of "expert" knowledge in the fields of, for example, immunology, neurology, and rheumatology. Prescriptions for pharmaceuticals, referrals to specialists, and diagnostic procedures are linked directly to *identifying* and *treating* specific diseases. Both public and private health insurance companies usually cover expenses related to diagnosis. However, the costs of treatment are only partially covered by insurance. Only those deemed appropriate methods to treat illness are paid for under most plans while alternative treatments are only partially covered or not covered at all, as for example, massage, naturopathic medicine, and physiotherapy.

This naming through diagnosis also contributes to individual and social understandings of ill bodies by attaching an accepted explanation of a chronically ill body that makes sense biomedically to a *specific* body. The diagnostic process as part of biomedical discourse is a primary method of legitimating ill bodies. The concrete practice of diagnosis involves examining the material body by testing bodily fluids, scrutinizing internal and external body parts, and recording chronologies of "subjective" experiences of feeling unwell. Once the body has been "fully" examined, a physician declares a disease category as an explanation of the deviation from a "normally" functioning body, in its idealized form. Underlying this process of examination are assumptions about what constitutes a healthy body and how the body is supposed to function. Operating from a stance that there is a relatively complete and precise knowledge about the body and how it functions provides a foundation from which biomedical practitioners can claim competence to judge what is illness and what is health.

Biomedical discourse is routinely reproduced through concrete practices associated with diagnosis. Because of this privileged stature of diagnosis in society more widely, if no disease process is "discovered" operating in a body or no illness declared as an "official" diagnosis, then that body becomes invalid *discursively*. There is no legitimate claim to illness and the individual's experience of illness may be subsequently dismissed and devalued by friends, family, coworkers, and medical practitioners.[1] One way to understand everyday experiences of women with chronic illness and the ways they negotiate their social and physical environments is to look at the process through which illness is made culturally intelligible through the practice of diagnosis. In other words, how does diagnosis contribute to marking women's chronically ill bodies so that they are read as (legitimately) ill bodies? For us, this involves scrutinizing meanings associated with both women and specific types of chronic illness and how they become attached to the women's chronically ill bodies. In the rest of this chapter, we draw out the discursive instability of the material body by using some of the women's experiences of the often long, drawn-out process of diagnosis for Myalgic Encephalomyelitis (ME), Rheumatoid Arthritis (RA), and associated illnesses. We first discuss "bodies in context" and the onset of illness. As the women's notions of illness and health destabilize, so too the women struggle to make discursive

sense of their continually destabilizing bodies. We then show how this destabilization finds interim fixities through the women's active role in discursively defining their bodies through ascribing labels of illness, with the
assistance of biomedical practitioners' diagnoses. We then turn to elaborating
in more detail specific bodily inscriptions, including the women's movements toward expressing their embodiment in ways that adjust these inscriptions so that they make sense within the women's own corporeal spaces.

ONSET

Onset of chronic illness varied from woman to woman. Nearly all of the
women diagnosed with RA as an adult could link onset of illness with a
stressful event—death of a partner, relationship breakup, birth of a child, or
a severe trauma. Onset as an event was so momentous in some of the wom-
en's lives that they could pinpoint an exact moment when they felt the disease take hold of a part of their body. For example, Noreen recounted how
she woke up with a sore ankle and thought she had twisted it without noticing the day before. As the day wore on, the pain in her ankle grew more
intense. By the end of the day, she could not even drag her foot to the car,
let alone drive home. Over the next few months, the pain, "like a blowtorch
emanating from deep within the skin," spread to other joints. Even though
it was clear that something was affecting her body, it was not until six
months later that a positive rheumatoid factor showed up in her blood and
the physician prescribed something that might arrest the pain.

Noreen's experience is not atypical of the other women in the study. Eve
experienced pain in her shoulder joints initially right after kayaking, and,
subsequently, on numerous occasions, she variously attributed the pain to
gardening, cycling, or driving. But after having slept 16 hours and awaken-
ing to immobile, swollen joints with no obvious activity to blame, she talked
with a physician. The physician was reluctant to consider RA. Once Eve
persisted in her claims of pain, fatigue, and swollen joints, her doctor recommended she see a rheumatologist, who immediately diagnosed RA.

Not all diagnoses come about so quickly. For some women, onset of illness takes place over a longer period of time, with less easily identifiable
symptoms, making the destabilization of the body all the more distressing.
In some instances, the women experienced a series of seemingly unrelated
bouts of illness, such as the flu, then a cold, followed by an injury, and then
an infection. Such a series of assaults on the body sets up a perplexing web
of destabilizations, which, when read collectively as one illness, produces in
some women a response of incredulity or impossibility. Nicola's experience
with a rare type of arthritis demonstrates that the experience of a series of

apparently disparate sets of recoverable illnesses diffuses the intensity of the recognition of the seriousness of a chronic illness.

Over a period of three to four years, Nicola struggled to recover from the initial viral assault on the body. She contracted the *Shigella* bacteria[2] somewhere on her travels. After a singular bout of dysentery-like symptoms, she recovered and continued traveling. Over the next year, she suffered a recurring series of infections—of the eye, ear, throat, and bladder—all of which were treated individually by different doctors in different countries with antibiotics. When aches and pains became the most prominent symptoms affecting her lifestyle, Nicola went to a rheumatologist, who diagnosed Reiter's Syndrome.[3] The physician prescribed steroids to arrest the progression of the disease. Once the physician reduced the dosage, Nicola stopped seeing her and eventually stopped taking the medication. Two years later, Nicola experienced a similar set of symptoms—infection after infection, aches on top of pains, specialist after specialist—in the end only to be re-diagnosed with Reiter's Syndrome.

The destabilization of her material body left Nicola in a state of intermittent worry with fluctuating abilities. She was in her late twenties and had not paid much attention to the materiality of her body, depending instead on its invincibility. When diagnosed the first time with Reiter's Syndrome, the disease made no impact discursively; she did not tell anyone of her illness nor did she get any more information about the illness beyond that which the physician passed along to her at the time. When diagnosed the second time, the collapse of her body had been more complete, that is, more bodily systems had broken down and the pain and fatigue interfered more extensively with her daily living activities. She learned more about the disease and found out that biomedical research had shown that when individuals suffering Reiter's Syndrome symptoms did muscle-building exercises during remission periods, flare-ups would not be as severe. She now wonders about her initial refusal of having a body with Reiter's Syndrome, or what we could call her refusal of the discursively ill body. Had she learned more about the illness, she might have realized that the disease recurs and that when the disease goes into remission she could have been preparing for the next bodily assault by doing bodybuilding exercises. She claims that had she paid attention the first time, she would not be suffering as much now.

Onset of illness for other women, rather than experienced as an initial assault followed by recurring attacks, bore the pattern of long-term, slowly developing, nagging sets of symptoms that were difficult to describe and even harder to make sense of. Many of the women experienced fleeting symptoms that could not easily be connected: a fall masked as a stumble over a water sewer grate, sore wrists explained by computer keyboard strain, or temporary blindness accounted for by auras associated with migraines. Rarely did the women describe this initial state of being, before words overpowered the experience with a specific meaning.

Yet there were a few women who pointed toward the existence of a pre-discursive ill body. For example, when Connie described the onset of ME after a particularly severe flu, she linked the feeling first to mental illness, then to being a "mass of mess."

> I couldn't breathe. There was, probably, a very, very, very, very gentle angle. I couldn't get to the back of the garden, to the back door and I see really how gentle that, I couldn't make it up that slope, that hill. And everything collapsed that day. [My husband] called me and said, "how are you doing," and I said "I'm mentally . . . I think, I'm mentally unbalanced." That's how I felt because I couldn't figure out the difference between anything. It just felt like I was just this mass of mess. I couldn't isolate a headache, I couldn't isolate the body, I couldn't isolate fatigue, I couldn't isolate pain, I couldn't isolate cold symptoms, you know, it was just a mass of mess.

In articulating her experience through this idea of being a "mass of mess," Connie comes close to describing what we would consider the pre-discursive ill body. During this collapse, Connie was not able to differentiate her own body from her immediate surroundings, either socially or physically. The disjuncture that Connie was feeling between her physical being and its placement in her garden could be explained as the jumble, clutter, and muddle of experiencing illness. Yet this ontological dissonance between what she was feeling and what she thought she was supposed to be feeling—expressed as mental illness—had already been coded as one of abnormality. In her struggle to come up with language to describe her experience, Connie chose to cast her mental faculties as lacking rather than her physical body as collapsing, perhaps reflecting that in being unable to give a name to such physical sensations, the only feasible explanation seemed to be one of impending madness.

For other women, illness did not make itself so readily known. Many women who depicted the onset of their illness as taking over a period of years tended to describe the onset as a loss of being able to do regular, everyday things. Gina, in her account of ME, described onset as

> Absolutely debilitating fatigue. Unable to, unable to brush my daughter's long hair. Unable to, my youngest daughter still needed help shampooing her hair and combing it out, and I was unable to do that. Unable to leave the house and do anything. Unable to read the newspaper. Unable to watch TV. But these were symptoms like those symptoms lasted for three years. The other one that was a pain, pain all over my body. Every muscle, every joint. And sleep. I could not, for the first six months of my illness, I could not keep awake. It was like I felt like I had narcolepsy. I was so tired, I could not go to

movies, I could not talk with people, I could not smile or laugh. Or, I was too sick. All I wanted to do was to be left alone. I always got up and got dressed every day. But I ended up on the sofa, and I thought it would just be temporary, and I ended up on the sofa for two years. And unable to do just the basics.

Not being *able* to do the "basics" sometimes was not enough to be taken seriously by physicians. For many of the women, what eventually was recognized as the onset of illness was initially disregarded or misdiagnosed. Ongoing symptoms masqueraded as another illness, sometimes chronic, sometimes acute, with women being told over and over again that there was no disease, and "it is only in your head." This was especially the case for women who eventually were diagnosed, like Reann, as having ME.

I had a whole slew of symptoms and, at the time, I didn't know I had any! And I was told it just was stress. I thought I was having heart attacks and was in the hospitals for chest pains. And then all of the other symptoms, the acute phase, things like memory loss, the night sweats, irritable bowel. I couldn't eat anything. You know, I was allergic to everything. And I think the memory loss was the worst. That's what I found was the final straw, is when I decided that I couldn't cope with working full time. Because I had taken a couple of extended leaves of absence, trying to figure out what was going on. I was too tired to work, just too tired.

Many women were told definitively that their symptoms were due to stress, so that they were left on their own, sometimes for years, to make sense of their own individual "masses of mess." For nearly all these women, there was a moment when they knew that something else was wrong, that it was not "just stress," that there was something systematic going on in their bodies, even if it were unpredictable.

DIAGNOSIS

Commonly women were anxious during the period between onset and diagnosis. Most of the anxiety arose out of not knowing what was wrong and not being able to control their bodies, their environments, and their lives. There was also the sense of not knowing what "it"—the unidentified disease process—could or could not do. Rhoda thought the RA diagnosis was scary for she didn't understand what "it" would do to her body. Charlotte was shocked and Helen did not understand why the doctor was so concerned. Noreen concluded quickly that the disease would shorten her life and was frightened about what the future held for her. Mary Ann, too, was scared.

I freaked. I just bawled. All I could think of was that it was—I was going to be crippled, because I just kept picturing old people where their joints are deformed and their hands and they use canes, and all the rest of it. And so I felt—first, it was disbelief. In fact, I demanded that I have an MRI done on my knees and my hands, because I thought there must be something that they're missing. There's no way that I have rheumatoid arthritis. And so, he said okay, and he set up the MRI. And then he said, once, you know, you get the results come back and see me. So I got—there was nothing showing on the MRI, just inflammation, and so it was just—I had to do that to tell my—to eliminate anything else. And then, so then when it was, that's what it has to be, it just—I couldn't believe it. He recommended that I go see the Arhritis Centre. And I was very thankful that I went there. First, when I went there I thought, oh, I'm just going to be in a room full of all these old people, who are going to be, you know, complaining, and this and that. And—I have a, I'm a very optimistic person, and although something's gone wrong in my system, I try and—okay, well, what can I do to help myself and that type of thing. So I went in this room, and they give you an information session on rheumatoid arthritis, about what it is and it was very informative . . . it was a great session. There were also two younger girls, both younger than myself. I was 29 at that time. And, so that was great to meet them, because we shared a lot of the same signs and symptoms, and I didn't feel so alone then.

Mary Ann refused to believe that RA could affect her body. Yet once she accepted that it might be a possibility and sought support, she temporarily stabilized her discursive body with the label of an illness. She also began shifting her image of what an arthritic body looks like so as to accommodate her own body into that discourse. Janet, previously athletic, had found the diagnosis frightening and dissonant with her image of herself and her knowledge of her body.

What in the heck did I do to deserve this? . . . I was just amazed at the swiftness of the disease's progression. And I guess just quite afraid. Fear was probably the biggie. Lying in bed at night. You know, you draw these pictures in your head about yourself as a disabled person. And you never in your wildest dreams thought that would be, you know, again, especially given my athletic background. And then coping with the loss of use of your body. Kind of going through that mourning period. You do mourn for parts of you that just aren't there anymore. And you are not able to rely on your own physical strength to do things yourself. Which is quite a challenge.

For both Mary Ann and Janet, along with the destabilization of their material bodies, came space for the negotiation of possible bodies that might "fit" their own experiences. Mary Ann found that space through interaction with other young women in a supportive environment, which began to dissolve images of old people, "crippled" with arthritis. For Janet, mourning specific body parts assisted her in moving toward a space where she could recognize herself as someone with RA instead of the physically fit, strong athlete.

While the diagnosis process for RA is relatively straightforward, this is not the case for ME. Diagnosis for ME is based on a process of elimination of other illnesses that have more conclusive, though still uncertain, lab tests. Approaching diagnosing an illness by eliminating other illness where there are no definitive tests slows down the process of diagnosis, particularly when there is the presence of symptoms associated with other diseases and illnesses, such as depression and lupus. Diagnosis of ME for the women in this study ranged from three months (Verna) to several years (Raquel [13], Stella [12], Teresa [13]) after contacting the family doctor to first discuss the symptoms. Many of the women were diagnosed with other illnesses before either ME or MS: Raquel with Myelodysplasia Syndrome; Janice with depression and chronic mononucleosis; and Jayne, Teresa, and Sophie, with depression; while Stella, Debby, and Dolores, though diagnosed, refused the label of depression. And Sandra was diagnosed with Multiple Sclerosis before settling with the disease label of ME.

No matter the diagnosis, nearly all of the women expressed a certain sense of relief when finally ascribed a label to the constellation of symptoms they were experiencing. For the women with RA, there was also the sense that they would now be able to gain some control over their symptoms through treatment. For women with ME, the response was more commonly one of "Oh, what's that?" The materiality of the disease process of RA is more prominent in popular knowledge than that of ME. Although the women diagnosed with RA came to know that there was potential for serious physical deterioration and incapacity, many expressed initial relief on diagnosis which provided an explanation for their symptoms. Gaining knowledge that the disease has an unpredictable course, but no cure, however, left women with considerable uncertainty. For women with ME, the relief associated with the diagnostic label of "ME" is exemplified by Agnes' comment.

> I was delighted, actually. I thought thank heavens, I've got a name for it. There is something the matter with me. I'm not going nuts. . . . I thought I had early Alzheimer's because the symptoms were so similar. I couldn't make change, I couldn't calculate, and in the back of my mind was how many times have I said to people well, can your mother make change? Does she have difficulty with accounts? I thought I can't make change, I do my bank book and I'll do it again. I couldn't remember phone numbers. I would look in the phone book for a phone number, but I learned there was no way I could close the book and dial the number, I had to keep it open, I had to keep my finger on it because the time I got around to dialing, I'd have forgotten it.

To have a label that indicates the illness is not of psychological origin vindicated many of the women's experiences of their bodies. A diagnosis of ME meant that there was some "cause" for the destabilization of the body; and once there was a "cause," there may be a "cure." Similarly, to have a label might mean that there are more systematic treatment regimes available. As we noted before, most of the women knew there was something askew in their physical body before this was accepted by biomedical practitioners. With a diagnositic label of RA or ME, they now had a discourse from which they could draw meaning, and perhaps physical relief.

DIAGNOSIS AS INSCRIPTION

Although women with chronic illness experience symptoms simultaneously as a "mass of mess," through diagnosis as a "naming" practice, the women are able to bring about a sense of unity to a particular configuration of symptoms. This unity, expressed as RA or ME for example, is a discursive category that is constitutive of the women's experiences of chronic illness. It is important to note that constitutive processes of a discursive category of a disease do not begin with an ascriptive label. Taking Chantal Mouffe's notion of the constitutive outside seriously means that the discursive categories of RA and ME have, up to the point, already been actively ascribed to healthy bodies—if only as one of absence. For example, a healthy body does not express the constellation of symptoms associated with the discursive categories of RA or ME; so, the body is inscribed as not-RA and not-ME. Many of the women illustrated this point when they contrasted their experiences of illness with their experiences prior to onset of symptoms. Pauline describes her abilities in the context of not being able to do the "basics."

> And the muscle weakness. A lot of muscle weakness. And very hard to concentrate, like, if I was watching television I could feel my eyes focusing, so I had a lot of vision problems, and I couldn't read. You know, there was this dyslexia. It was interesting. I'd read—I look at something, and I couldn't—I could read, but by the time I got to the end of the sentence I didn't know what the first of the sentence was about. So there was mostly the . . . you know, I felt well enough to sort of be up. It was the cognitive—I felt it was the cognitive problems that were the most startling. . . . And then I couldn't even go—a lot of muscle weakness, like, I couldn't comb my hair, or, you know, if I'd comb my hair I had to use, you know, sort of use this arm to hold the . . .

What is interesting in Pauline's discussion of her body is the implicit assumption that a body without ME could accomplish these tasks with ease, relying on the smooth functioning of the brain, and without even noticing specific movements of body parts—her eyes, hands, and arms. Yet at the point of the ascription of the diagnosis as a discursive category, the women are put into the position of having to deal with the surfacing of some of the unspoken assumptions defining ill and healthy bodies.

For women with chronic illness, dealing with discourses that have been involved in the social practices of "naming" symptoms and diagnosis entails drawing meaning from them to make sense of their daily living spaces. One process through which women come to embody illness is through *inscription*—the etching onto the body a particular rendering of an idealized or fleshed body. Through inscription of several discourses, including the ones involved in ascribing a diagnosis, women with chronic illness come to be *specific* bodies. This involves a process that constitutes the body as culturally intelligible—to others and to the women themselves. Women may also attempt to reinscribe, and so respecify, their bodies in resistance to an inscription that challenges their identity or position as a valued person. First, in this process, is a surface inscription onto a passive body.[4] Here the body is a surface upon which laws, morality, and values about health and illness are either visibly or invisibly inscribed through rituals, social practices, and medical procedures. Second is an internalized mapping of a socially negotiated discourse. Here embodiment, the being of a bodily form and its social constructions, is constituted through the internalization of "normal" and "natural" notions of ill, diseased, and healthy bodies. Third is what we term *reinscription* as a resistance strategy. Here the body and embodiment are rewritten, or reinscribed, through specific sets of bodily activities that counter the hegemonic discourses of illness, disease, and health. These sets of bodily activities filter the idealized body through the destabilized/destabilizing body.

Surface Inscriptions

Surface inscriptions, like the ones we have discussed thus far, are closely linked to shifts in ability and image. For women diagnosed with severely degenerating types of arthritis, images of older, "crippled" bodies became part of their notion of what RA or Reiter's Syndrome *could do* to their bodies. These visible images are augmented by other visible markers of "crippling" illness, as for example, metal and plastic wrist, arm, and knee braces; canes, walkers, and other assistive devices; and wheelchairs and scooters for mobility. These reminders "mark" the body as somewhat deviant, abnormal, and disabled, so that the body under these circumstances can be read effortlessly in a straightforward manner by others encountered in everyday life, such as bus drivers, store clerks, physicians, and friends.

Bringing the body and, in particular, body parts into the purview of medicine facilitates a palpable manifestation of a surface inscription through removal, replacement, or an addition of a body part. Several of the women with RA had joints replaced—Belle, Bette, Margie, and Sara. We consider these literal, sub-surface inscriptions whereby the disease category of arthritis is inscribed physically into the body—initially visibly through bandages and assistive devices and later invisibly by covering up any scars left by incisions.

With these types of inscriptions, the discursive category of illness emerges only when details about the joint replacement become known, usually through some sort of revelation in conversation or through information solicited on a medical form. Like a diagnosis, the discursive category of "joint replacement" legitimates to a certain extent a woman's previous experience of pain and immobility among friends, family, and acquaintances.

Surface inscriptions were quite common among the women we talked with. As we have discussed so far, women with arthritis tended to focus on the materiality of disease inscriptions—what their bodies would look like in a few years—whereas women with ME tended to wrap themselves up in refusing discursive categories, particularly those associated with illness with psychological origins. Dolores and Vivienne vehemently refused the discursive inscription of depression, both referring to notions of "slacking." Dolores had been employed as a nurse for a long time before onset of illness. In addition to muscle weakness, cognitive impairment and memory loss impeded her ability to remain employed. Her physician diagnosed depression and told her that she was "just slacking off" and that "he had many patients that would love to go work." She continually maintained that she was neither depressed nor slacking. Her feelings of being "down in the dumps" stemmed directly from not being able to practice nursing. Linking depression with "slacking" is a powerful way to recast the feeling of lethargy—which is often linked to depression and ME—with a socially devalued behavior.

For Vivienne, the image of a "slacker" was equivalent to having an irresponsible work ethic. While growing up, family members, except for her mother, all had a "strong work ethic," putting in long hours of paid work then spending the majority of their spare time engaging in physical sport. The family, collectively, had always viewed the mother as a "slacker" because she needed much rest and did not work long hours in either paid or unpaid work.[5] With the onset of ME, which for Vivienne was an acute episode of a flu-like virus, she struggled to keep at bay the inscription of "slacker"—by not telling her family she was ill and pushing herself physically even after her collapse.

The women with ME did not refuse all discursive categories, however. In fact, most women actively sought out a diagnosis that they could claim as their own so that they could contribute to reinscribing their body as one that was legitimately ill. As Dolores and Vivienne show, it was not just any diagnosis that would be useful for reinscription. For women with ME, depression leaves a negative, belittling impression because the description of illness does not encompass what it is they feel, either emotionally or physically. They continued to seek a diagnosis that would describe both, even if this meant they would have to change doctors, take more tests, or even prompt the specialist to consider a different disease altogether. Leeza described this process in detail.

I think about two years after it started, then, because nobody knew what I had, I mean nobody in church knew what I had, nobody in the community. I didn't know. The doctors didn't know. So finally a friend had found this magazine article, and she said, that sounds like you. So she gave me a copy of it, and I read it and I thought, yeah, that sounds like me. So in there it actually talked about a test that you could find out whether you had it or not. So I took that to my doctor, and said, well, you know, could I have this test taken. And she said, yes, that would be fine. But she said we still can't do anything for you. So I said, well, at least I'll know what I have. You know, I mean even that is kind of nice, you know, I mean, you go and talk with people, and well, what's your problem? Right? I mean, you look fine, so why aren't you out there doing things? So she took this . . . test, and it came back positive. So—but at that time it was called the Epstein-Barr virus—actually the Chronic Epstein-Barr Virus Syndrome they were calling it at that time. So that's what she said, that, that [I had].

Attaining an "appropriate" category was one way the women could influence the circumstances within and through which their own sets of activities would constitute their experience of being ill. By taking on the discursive category of ME, the women could thwart the negative connotations associated with depression as well as other psychosomatic interpretations of their symptoms and take up a competing marker that would permit them to present their symptoms as part of a different, physically and socially justifiable set of experiences.[6]

Internalized Inscriptions

Alongside these surface inscriptions are internal mappings of what it is like to be ill. The invisibility of many of these surface inscriptions were complicated by the invocation of these internalized inscriptions by people the women interacted with as well as by the women themselves. What the women did not anticipate was that indeterminacy of chronic illness would be compounded by allying themselves with a biomedically contested discursive disease category (a theme we discuss more thoroughly in chapter 8). The "justifiability" of ME as a physically and socially legitimate illness was often questioned by family, friends, coworkers, medical professionals, and even by the women themselves, calling upon the women to produce "evidence" that they were indeed ill over and over again. Shelagh makes this point in her story of running into a friend at a restaurant during the time she was on sick leave from work.

[A]nd people say, well you look great. And somehow I'm sure they are not saying that but you feel they are saying, well then, what's the matter with you? [Said in a sarcastic tone.] [If] I had casts or deformed arms, then they would go, how are things going, Shelagh? [Said in a patronizing tone.] Because you look all right then think, it's very, it's like a silent, invisible disease and I mean it's hard enough for yourself to understand that I can understand it is very hard on other people to figure out while you're walking. I ran into [a friend] the one day and he goes, "Oh, yeah, sure, you're sick." Because if you are sick you are home all of the time and you can't go out for supper.

Shelagh identified the key component of legitimating an ill body socially—one has to look ill to be ill. What illness looks like can vary. Shelagh, like many of the women with arthritis, appealed to a disfigured body as an (idealized) image of illness. But illness can also comprise a dazed look, slurred words, listless facial expressions, jittery hand movements, and incoherent speech. What is problematic for women with invisible chronic illness, especially ME, is that the woman's body must be filtered through an internalized notion of what a "normal" body is. Alice's family thought she was faking illness, probably for attention. Her family's reaction to caring for her sister with cancer showed Alice that family members were not interested in having ill relatives. When she gained weight, they made fun of her—for if she were not ill, then her weight gain could only indicate "slacking off" and laziness. In normalizing discourses about health, illness, ability, and disability, whether or not the illness is visible matters for women with chronic illness in the sense of *how* a woman with chronic illness is or may be devalued and dismissed.

Visibility of illness is not the only theme running through the women's experiences of normalizing discourses. Naturalizing the notion of health and ability entails normalizing illness and disability, too: there are prescriptive norms of what it is to be "normally" ill, trotted out as a "blueprint" when dealing with a potentially ill woman. Normalizing illness, as another way to filter an idealized body with a destabilized one, only in this case the idealized body is the one which is ill, is an example of the second type of inscription we identified, an internal mapping of a socially negotiated discourse. Social practices associated with normalizing discourses about bodies discipline the body from an early age, defining what it means to be healthy and ill, and what it means to be "normal" and "deviant." Ronnie, who was diagnosed with RA as a child, knew that she was not "normal" even though her illness was never openly discussed. That there was a normal body against which she was being judged was never in question; that she was abnormal had always been assumed. For Belle, who was also diagnosed with RA as a child, normality was constantly at the forefront of interaction with other people because the damage to her joints was visible from an early age. Although body image was not prominent in Belle's negotiation of discourse around health and ability, body image is integral to normalizing discourses. There is a rejection of disabled (and disfigured) bodies as part of any idealized lifestyle.

Some women struggled to resist normalizing illness and refused inscriptions of certain notions of illness. Brie was so successful at hiding her illness publicly, she shocked her employer when she finally quit due to illness. For Julia and Janet, not being cast as deviant meant continuing to lead "normal" lives. For both women, normality was rooted in maintaining employment.

> I pretty much just went to work and went home, 'cause I didn't want to lose that link with normal life—which was the job! I was afraid of, uhm, getting devoured by it. So I, that's why I thought the best thing is let all the other things slide, and just go to work, make sure that I keep myself relatively together, just so that I can go to work. [Julia]

> [The illness is] just something beside me. I didn't want to take it on and have it become a real part of who I am. And working, continuing to work, continuing to go to the gym, even though it was painful was still the way of, oh, I'm sure some people would call it denial. But for me it was just maintaining as much of my "normal life" as I could. And staying at work was a big part of that. [Janet]

Hanging onto "normality" meant resisting any inscription as ill and deviant, leading a "normal(ized)" life, and sustaining a public image of health, strength, and fitness. Although Julia was diagnosed with ME and Janet with RA, both were successful in hiding their illness, at least for a time, which enabled them to remain publicly inscribed as healthy and normal.

The articulation of other discourses that influence the negotiation of notions of being ill, as for example, motherhood, work, and beauty, have played out in distinctive ways among the women we talked with. Part of the difficulty for Gina with being ill had been that she could not fulfill her expectations of "normal" activities, even the basic tasks of motherhood, like combing her daughter's hair. Not only did she see herself as failing at being healthy, she also saw herself as failing at being a mother. Ruth saw herself as being lazy rather than ill because she could not complete the simplest set of work tasks set out for her: "It's like the anorexic. They look in the mirror and they see fat. I look in the mirror and I see lazy, you know?" Interestingly, she draws on another contested illness, anorexia nervosa, to make the point that it is not only conceptions of weight that women internalize, but also notions of activity: if you are not active and out doing things, then you are lazy, and, consequently, a "bad" person. Furthermore, links were made by some women between activity, disability, and sexuality. Mary Ann, for example, was in her late twenties when she was diagnosed with RA. She was sensitive to the possibility that physical disability would interfere with her attractiveness as a heterosexual woman.

> I was in a relationship at the time when I went to the [information] session. I came home, I went over to this—my boyfriend's house, and I was talking with

him. And we were having dinner and I was talking about this session. And he
said, you know, it's really strange to be talking about arthritis. Like, who talks
about arthritis over dinner. And he just couldn't deal with it, like, our relationship never worked, because he couldn't deal with that. You know. And that
was pretty traumatic too, because I felt, my God, everyone's going to judge
me because I have this disease going on in my system, right? And that's a pretty
traumatic thing, as well. Mind you, they're not worth having in your life if
they're that type of person. So I was glad I learned that about him.

Like Mary Ann, after onset and diagnosis of chronic illness, the women
were forced to negotiate the material limits of the body with internalized
discursive inscriptions, the latter most often expressed as "society's expectations." The women, of course, did not deal with one expectation at a time.
Akin to feeling like a "mass of mess" upon the destabilization of the material
body, the women experienced a battery of expectations at the same time,
filtering them through their destabilized/destabilizing body. Eve described
her feelings of being overwhelmed by a "mass of expectations."

I think that society has taught us to have extremely high expectations of ourselves. The things I do, I can't say I do, because [no one] is watching me or
grading me. Or, it's just that I figure that it's my job to do all these things.
And I've had to do a lot of thinking about that since, when you get hit with
something like this [RA] you have to adjust your thinking all about. And I
think that I am supposed to be a super-terrific mom. I'm supposed to be out
there on the soccer field every Saturday. I am supposed to have the house all
clean and the garden freshly planted. And gourmet summer cooking for nice
friends on Saturday night. And professionally capable and professionally
clothed. And good with my hands and capable of fixing things around here.
And sometimes it blows my head off, all the things that I think I am supposed
to do. And most of them I can do. But you can't do them and maintain your
health when you have something like this. Actually I don't think women,
period, can do all those things and maintain their health. When you throw in
life's crooks, you know, and all of a sudden you are suffering from a disease,
or your child is suffering from something, or your parent is ill, or financial
hardships. You add anything extra to all those things that you are already
doing, you are just a waiting time bomb. And I know that when I get into my
mode of trying to get everything perfect, everything together, then so I can
relax—that's how I can relax—is when everything else is all done. That's when
I think that if anything disturbs that, or adds to it, that's when I'll blow.

Eve did not elaborate what she meant by "blow," but what we can surmise
is that this describes the point at which she can no longer maintain the façade
of "holding it all together"—the disjuncture between discourse and materiality would be far too great. By "blowing," she reintegrates her modified physi-

cal being with a modified set of expectations, or, what we might say, she comes to recognize her embodiment.

Recognizing embodiment, in this case through transferring the limits of the material body to various notions of being a mother, a worker, and a life partner, invites palpable interpretations of the inscriptions of illness. The women tended to portray their illness initially, both in their narratives and during the course of their illness, in either/or terms, and then completed their depictions by associating their ill bodies as part of the negative side of the dualism. As the women talked more and as the women were ill longer, they tended to portray the complexities of their illness in terms of both/and. For example, Gina explains her impressions of another woman's narrative of illness at a support group session she had attended when first diagnosed with ME.

> And I went to my first meeting and the woman I sat beside, I asked her how long she had had this illness. Now this was, I had just had it for six months, I'd been newly diagnosed. I was on the sofa all day, so I could rest up, so I could have the energy to go to the meeting. I went to the meeting and I asked her how long she had had it. And she said eleven years. And I just, I started to cry. Because I can't live like this for eleven years. There is no way. I cannot lie on the sofa for eleven years and not have a life. And what I didn't find out until through the meeting is that she had been really sick for three years and had gotten a lot better and was working full time and had worked all day that day and had walked to the meeting, which was about a mile or something from her house. But she didn't tell me that. And she had sort of leftover symptoms, but she was functional.

At the time of the meeting, Gina was in the midst of her first collapse, where the physical symptoms of the illness overwhelmed any thought about being either ill or healthy. Yet during that meeting, Gina realized that this woman was indeed ill, but she was also functioning pretty well—she was *both* ill *and* healthy. This kind of insight is enormously useful in support group situations. Women with ME can begin to negotiate the discursive category of illness and include their own bodily experiences into the sets of bodily activities they engage in. Janice, when under pressure from her family to accept that her symptoms were psychological and not physiological, understood her body quite differently: "You are either sick and you can't work, or you're not sick. Where what I was hoping for was to get compensation for the amount that I wanted to work but wasn't able to." Her experience of bodily limits spurred her to reformulate what accommodation in the workplace actually means—facilitating a *specific* environment for *specific* bodies, bodies and environments that are embodied.

Reinscription as Resistance

Challenging the fixity of discursive categories opens up space not only to
negotiate discursive categories, but also to engage in rewriting the body with
and through competing renditions of what it is to be ill and what it is to be
healthy. Many of the women engaged in re-sorting their living circumstances
as a way to contest the predominance of specific interpretations of illness,
health, or disability. Thus far, we have discussed some of the ways the
women resisted a diagnosis of being ill, but we have not shown how women
reinscribed their bodies with competing notions of illness, health, ability,
and disability. Some of the women were able to reinsert themselves into the
process of producing meanings of chronic illness and of disability by drawing
on their own experiences and by writing "normality" over illness, somewhat
like donning a protective suit of armor forged from dominant social norms
and mores.

The women's reinscriptions met with mixed success. For example, Teresa
sought out information from four different local support groups, each associated with an ME symptom. She came to terms with her ill body by isolating
a symptom—pain, agoraphobia, malaise, and anxiety—and using each to
connect with a network of other people, most often by telephone, a socially
acceptable way to interact. Similarly, Yvonne isolated her symptoms, yet
instead of connecting with other people through articulating her ill body,
she sought to isolate her body and moved into a sterile environment, a new
suit of armor. Through assistance from family members, she was able to
revamp a house to accommodate her severe allergies. Rather than hiding illness, like Brie, Julia, and Janet did, some of the women renegotiated what it
meant to be ill. For example, Bette, in resisting the inscription of RA as a
disabling chronic illness, used her car and her dress as ways to inscribe normality onto her ill body. Bette connects her own mobility to her car—
"There's no where I can't go. . . . [I]f I didn't have a car and I wasn't able
to drive, I don't think I would be very happy." Having access to a car assists
Bette in transforming the image of RA as disabling to one where RA is sec-
ondary to negotiating the city. Even though the disease process restricts her
bodily movement, she is able to overcome household confinement by being
able to drive. The car itself acts as a suit of armor protecting Bette from an
externally inscribed disabled body.

Dress, too, assists Bette in reinscribing her body as "not disabled." For
Bette, it is "very important" to appear in public wearing outfits with "everything matching." Clinging to and acting out a set of prescribed social behaviors permits Bette to claim "normality" without having to explain illness or
disability for she appears "normal," herself, like everyone else her age, even
though most people know she is ill. Like the car, socially appropriate cloth-
ing acts as a suit of armor, protecting her from what she considers public

disclosure of being disabled. Interestingly, these "normalizing" means are unstable for as she ages and as the disease progresses, her suits of armor begin failing. She recounted how she is beginning to feel out of place, not because of a more pronounced limp or an uneven gait (from her joint replacements), but because she increasingly can only wear sneakers. And, if she were to have to give up driving for health or financial reasons, as part of a set of bodily activities she engages in defining being "not disabled," the inscription of "normal" mobility would be shattered. Bette's uneasiness with her approach to being ill underscores the precariousness of reinscription in light of a fluctuating body.

This is not to say that reinscriptive processes as resistance only involve challenging normalizing discourse. The chronicity of illness and its unpredictability, both in the short and long term, appear to be key issues about the illness that the women deal with. Some women reinscribe their bodies through a sense of acceptance that they either have an ill body or they themselves are ill. We make this distinction between having an ill body and being ill here because there are ontological differences in the way women see themselves after onset and diagnosis of illness. Some women conceived of "having a chronic illness" as heightening the sense of the uncertainty of illness. Being sick is momentary but being ill is long-lasting. "Having an ill body" seemed like a delineation of illness in terms of body parts that are sick. This latter rendition is a common pain control strategy that women use, and are routinely taught in institutionalized settings. Either way, acceptance of having an illness or having a chronically ill body opens up the possibility of counterhegemonic inscriptions. Vivienne's eventual acceptance of being chronically ill shows how reinscription can rejuvenate one's ability to cope with being ill. She conceives the reinscription process as ongoing and distinguishes between the point of knowing about illness and understanding it. When talking about a sympathetic homeopath, Vivienne depicted someone who understood the illness as embodied.

Don't berate yourself that you're tired. If you're tired, go to sleep. You know? Don't start kicking yourself about why you shouldn't be tired, you know? If you're tired, go to sleep. Don't fight it. So that kind of an understanding [from others] and a changing in my thinking helped. . . . And it's, that's just a very, you know, learning to love yourself a bit more [approach], I think. About caring. About that, instead of telling myself how I should be feeling and behaving. . . . As a matter of fact the doctor that diagnosed said, you know, if I hadn't been so fit and into as much fitness I probably wouldn't have got sick sooner with something less severe; you know, there's a bit of a sad irony in that. You know, we're told that we're supposed to be fit and be out exercising all the time and all these and it's not a 100% true. . . . I think exercise is still really important but in moderation and now I'm learning to pay attention to how my body feels and what I can—what's reasonable and what's going to fatigue

me, what's going to be beneficial to me and so I'm gauged by that and instead
of saying well, if I'm into walking or back into running that I should be running 20 minutes or half an hour everyday or every other day, you know, having
a regimen, it's more like you know, paying attention to how I'm at now and
how it's feeling and now I know. . . . I have to be smarter and really respect
what my body is telling me because I tend to easily drive myself without paying
attention to that [inaudible] but so the exercise, um, and I just sort of take like
deep breaths but creating space for me.

Vivienne is redefining what it is to be ill in terms of redefining what it is to
be healthy. By shifting the notion that illness means collapsing, she is able
to de-link the discourse of being ill and rearticulate herself as being healthy.
In her example of the homeopath telling her to go to bed when she is tired,
she is reinscribing illness onto her body. Rather than linking her activity of
going to bed early, or in the middle of the day, to behavior of an ill person,
she redefines the activity as one of the behavior of a healthy person who
knows when it is time to rest. This type of reinscription reinvents what it is
to be ill by resisting the normalization of illness and altering the meanings
associated with specific activities.

In rewriting their bodies, Vivienne and women like her appropriated
familiar scripts, like that of health, and re-worked them to make them apply
to *their* experiences of *their* bodies. This reinscriptive process involved de-
linking chronic illness from its regularized, normalized, and naturalized
meanings and re-linking illness to more evocative, enabling, and notable
meanings. By notable, we mean those meanings that make the new inscription more meaningful for the women's *specific* bodies, and their embodiment, and more useful in terms of social and political activity. In addition to
Vivienne's experience of reconfiguring "health," women with chronic illness
sometimes reconfigure what it is to be disabled. For example, rather than
conceiving a body ravaged with Rheumatoid Arthritis as deformed and disabled, some women, like Belle, took on a new script that rewrote her body
as differently shaped and differently abled. Or another woman, Ronnie, with
an experience similar to Belle's, rewrote her body as unpredictably abled and
sometimes limited. The type of difference these women are referring to is
like the type of difference that Abigail Bray and Claire Colebrook define as
"positive" difference—an act of self-formation, which when seen "as positive, then the ethical value of an act is determined by evaluating its force
within a network of other acts and practices, and not in reference to a putative origin."[7] Even though they discuss sexual difference, we can apply a
modified version of their argument here in this context: constituting illness
and disability as the negation of health and ability for women with chronic
illness needs to be turned around to question the primacy of invoking
notions that determine whether a body is deformed, disabled, or sporadically

malfunctioning rather than engaged in a set of activities that are self-forming. Any difference that emanates from the interaction between the materiality of the body and its discursive categories can be seen as merely different from one another and not different from an idealized conception of what a body should be, that is, one that is shapely, able, and smoothly functioning.

DISCOURSE AND THE MATERIAL BODY

Intersections among various discourses and the destabilization of the material body are complexly interwoven through the experiences of women with chronic illness. Women draw out meaning of their bodies through ideas, notions, and words as part of the multiple discourses that constitute their experiences. These ideas and expectations become concretely tied to the body through the process of inscription—the discursive or material etching of a particular rendition of an idealized or fleshed body. These inscriptions, surface, internalized, or rooted in resistance, are fragile, unsteadily fixed, and open to new possibilities of ever-evolving meaning. Yet women with chronic illness seek out discursive categories through which to make sense of their fluctuating bodies and experiences of an unpredictable disease process. Even with the fluidity of inscriptions, the women find some solace in being able, at least temporarily, to "fix" their body discursively, the utility of which gives texture to their lived spaces, a theme we take up in the next chapter. Although these inscriptions can be as devastating as the physical sensations of illness, they are also significant in shaping the way in which the women respond to the ongoing fluctuations of their material bodies. No inscription is complete. Any discursive category etches contradictory renderings of idealized and fleshed bodies creating room for resistance and counterhegemonic *self*-inscriptions. Elizabeth Grosz questions the possibility of a truly autonomous self-inscription, something to which we would agree.[8] But the self-inscription we discuss here—in the form of reinscription as resistance—is not autonomous in the sense of a self-authoring subject;[9] rather, self-inscription takes place in the crevices of the incomplete hegemony of a discursive category, emerging in context from contradiction and paradox, and is as incomplete as any other inscription. This coincides with holding in tension the specificity of the body through a woman's embodiment. What makes reinscription conceived this way such a relevant activity for women with chronic illness is that they are able to reassert themselves as they *are*, in their indeterminable state of being, through their embodiment.

7

❦

Limits to the Body: Inscription, Income Issues, Borders

This isn't going so badly. I've made it through one class and one meeting. Only one more of each. I wonder what the principal wants. She'll want feedback on the new course design. That's probably it. And I have time to mark these last few papers. . . . Maybe Sujata is right. Maybe I should stick with naturopathy and forget biomedicine altogether. "Sure, I'll have tea. Only a little milk. Thanks." *Now that I'm sitting down. I can hardly move. That shoulder. It's sticking. Ouch! I've got to stop moving that. How much longer do I have to go on like this? . . . Does anyone else notice? They must. Why else would Silas pour me tea? I thought I was able to hide this "thing." Go about my business. Who else knows? . . . Why does it bother me so? No! She surely wouldn't call me in to tell me that I have to quit. Would she? Could she do that? No, she wouldn't do something like that. I should probably phone the union and ask about having to leave work. I wish I had thought about this when I went part-time. I don't want to lose my benefits. . . . Maybe this afternoon, we'll sit in a circle. That should help a bit. I'll be able to rest a little while the students are talking. . . . That hurts. What is this "thing"? It's in my body. But it's not like a broken bone that heals. When will it heal? This can't be normal? It's like a war going on and I'm the one left in chaos. Chaos. What a great word. . . . There. I'm done with these papers. I should really find a way to mark without having to write so much. Those days my hands hurt. . . . I need to get "smarter" about my work . . . in lots of different ways.*

Chronic illness, with its inherent fluctuations, undermines the expected stability of the material body. We understand the expected stability of the material body to be part of that which is taken-for-granted, that which enables women, for example, to cross their legs, eat cookies, and plan events.

105

Effects of a disruption at this fine scale of movement or functioning reverber-
ates throughout the rest of the body and affects the ways in which women
with chronic illness negotiate their immediate physical surroundings.
Because women with chronic illness cannot always rely on their bodies to do
what they want them to do at any given moment, plans beyond "the next
little while" become problematic. Pain, fatigue, difficulties with mobility,
and inconsistency of motor control limit the women's bodies physically. Sensations of pain may hinder a woman's plan to shop for groceries, experiences
of spatial disorientation may prevent a woman's desire to drive to visit a
friend, or feelings of embarrassment may hold back a woman from eating
out. The physicality of the illness tends to close off spaces presumed to be
accessible to them and consequently to bound a woman's corporeal space to
her immediate surroundings.

Understanding how these physical sensations affect the lives of women
with chronic illness prompts us to scrutinize these bodily limits in terms of
both the discourse and materiality of borders. Being able to negotiate discursive inscriptions of the body, as we discussed in the previous chapter, assists
in making sense of the "mass" of meanings ascribed to the body of a woman
with chronic illness. Women indeed challenge inscriptions, and poke at the
parameters of the fixity of meaning for specific chronic illnesses. We are also
interested in how to make sense of the material parameters in the daily lives
of women with chronic illness. These material parameters, which both
restrict and enable women to do certain things, include the ways women
with chronic illness negotiate their social and physical environments.[1] The
unpredictability of fatigue associated with ME, for example, can upset social
plans. What makes this problematic for the woman is that if she cancels too
many times, friends may simply stop phoning, further shrinking a woman's
already limited social environment. Or not being able to navigate a set of
steps may close off access to a friend's home and some public spaces. Examining the materiality of the spaces women with chronic illness traverse gives
us a fuller understanding of how chronic illness becomes constitutive of
women's identities. As well, how women arrange their living space in order
to accomplish a set of tasks while fatigued or in pain is important in figuring
out what living with chronic illness is like.

Deciding whether to defer to these limits of the body, framed as discursive
and material borders in our account here, influences decisions women with
chronic illness make with regard to the way they secure income and interact
with professionals to treat illness. As we have already noted, materiality in
our framework includes economic matters. These material limits are some of
the most obvious ones the women discussed, as for example, refusal of disability benefits, high costs of alternative therapies, and financial dependence
on men. The materiality of bodily limits also influenced choices about which
health regime to follow, which health care practitioner to see, and which

therapy to try next. Encountering these limits hastened the women's desires to "fix" what was "wrong" with their bodies and to find a "cure" for what ailed them.

Along with these specific sets of actions are scripts associated with their choices. The legitimacy of claiming an illness for their chronically ill bodies is closely linked to biomedicine, for without a diagnosis, other institutions (for example, workplaces, insurance companies, and government) are without an authoritative discourse to define a body as ill or in need of accommodation. While striving for legitimacy, women with chronic illness endeavor, at the same time, to find meaning of their illness outside the confines of a discourse of health and illness. For example, women with chronic illness may focus on personal development. Although this could be explained in part by women reacting to hegemonic notions of chronic illness in women as personal "failings,"[2] most of the women engaging in these activities saw them as a means to a more fulfilling life than that being presented to them in their material lives.[3] The concreteness of illness experienced through discursive and material inscriptions of their bodies was minimized and became more containable and limited as they made efforts to construct more ethereal notions of illness. Shifting the meaning of health and disability away from the materiality of the body enabled the women to restructure their corporeal spaces from ones of predominantly restrictive closure to sites largely for rejuvenation.

The experience of bodily limits with particularized scripts of illness can sometimes invalidate the materiality of the body. This invalidation manifests in a wide range of activities in a number of places, including the home, workplace, and other public places, as well as financially through potential loss of income and denial of disability benefits. In looking in detail at women's accounts of their experiences of chronic illness, it becomes clear that these bodily limits, conceived as material and discursive borders, are fluctuating, shifting, and permeable. This ongoing fluidity of borders creates room for negotiation and resistance of dominant readings of ill bodies, as well as of their social and physical environments. In the rest of this chapter, we explore the uneven destabilization of bodily limits that the women we talked with experienced throughout the course of their illness. We focus on the women's embodiment as a way to sort through the materiality of inscriptions and the physicality of illness. We then consider the impact of material borders within the women's corporeal spaces. This discussion leads into looking at, in more detail, the daily routines of women with chronic illness in order to be able to discern the intricacies of the impact of chronic illness on the meanings and use of women's immediate environments. We then turn to the wider issues of economic matters. Finally, we pull these fluid accounts together to show how these bodily limits are constitutive of permeable borders, borders that women with chronic illness exist within and negotiate in their social and physical environments.

INSCRIPTION

In the previous chapter, we discussed how various discursive inscriptions shaped women's experiences of chronic illness. Resisting these inscriptions was very much part of the women's negotiating the ascription of meaning. In complicating such notions of chronic illness, discourse around what counts as disability is unsettled. Women with chronic illness exist in between discourses of ability and disability, not fitting into one or the other. Within discourses of disability, whether in the sense of populist images or official definitions, because of the focus on the material body in defining what it is to be disabled, the materiality of the body is heightened. Women with chronic illness are often excluded in definitions of disability because policies have been consistently based on a definition rooted in the social model of disability. Not surprisingly, women with chronic illness experience the disabling aspects of their material body differently than those women. As with women not fitting normative images of being ill, disability also exists within the hegemonic notion of a "disabled body" or a "person with disabilities." Women with chronic illness tend to be marginalized within dominant notions of disability. Jeannette makes this point in her discussion of her negotiating the label of "disability" to fit her own experiences with RA.

And in a lot of ways, I think a lot of the focus on disability tends to be, very visible disabilities, with people who are, you know, in very obvious ways, constrained or limited and need to be accommodated with chairs or devices. And if you don't fit that category, you tend not be able to see yourself as legitimately belonging to that group. And, I mean, I really struggle with that. I think what I find most depressing is that attitude that everybody should be able-bodied, and if you are not, you still can achieve if you really want to. You know we have, have, you know who's the man who went across the country?

Interviewer: Rick Hansen?

That Rick Hansen idea of, you know, anybody can achieve. And I feel like saying, oh, fuck off, you know? It's not like that. You can't achieve. You are, your life is not the same. And, sometimes I think, you know, coming back to school and that, I can't have the same expectations as some people. And I mean, in a way, that might sound defeatist, but, on the other hand, I look at them and I think, why is it that able-bodiedness has to be the standard and that success on their terms has to be success on my terms. Why do I have to think in terms of what career am I going to get after this? I consider it just amazing that I am even going to be at university in some ways. And I look at that challenge, and I think, I don't know, I don't know how my health is going to be in five years. I don't know if I am going to be able to use what I'm doing now in what is considered [to be] a traditionally constructive way. You know? And sometimes my doctors say things like, well, how will you use this if you are having [symptoms of RA].

Jeannette is making two arguments here that speak directly to normalizing processes within disability discourse. First, she is challenging the monolithic notion of what it is to be disabled. She refuses to be cast as an impaired body caught up in the same expectations of able-bodiedness. She uses Rick Hansen as an exemplar of the view that the material limits of the body can be overcome by individual will and determination, personality characteristics popularly valued. Rick Hansen, a premier wheelchair athlete and paraplegic since fifteen, wheeled "around the world" in the mid-1980s. His achievements, beyond what most able-bodied people do, are what Jeannette finds to be the hegemonic norm against which she, as a disabled woman, is compared. She wants to claim more space for defining disability in terms of the chronicity of the disease. Second, in building upon the notion of chronicity, she identifies the absence of the discursive category of chronic illness in commonly understood trajectories of professional careers. By questioning her return to school after having raised children while being ill, she begins to destabilize her discursive body as one that is incapable of having a career. Because chronic illness is unpredictable, Jeannette cannot count on her body to be consistent enough to finish school, let alone pursue a career. Jeannette, in struggling against the normalizing processes, demonstrates how women with chronic illness encounter the limits to their material body.

Challenging the discursive inscriptions of limits to the material body can involve very specific acts. Some women are able to subvert the hegemony of a normative discourse on disability, and its commonsense associations, by openly contesting the definition of disability. Belle, for example, has had RA since she was a toddler. On occasion, she said she uses a wheelchair while shopping or taking public transit. When she notices that someone is either staring or talking about her because she is in a wheelchair, she stands up, throws her arms in the air, and shouts, "My god, I can walk again!" This disruption breaks the pattern of thinking about women in wheelchairs as being incapable of walking and subverts the more ominous inscription of walking being an indicator of able-bodiedness. Belle's simple act destabilizes discourse around disability, because she draws on popular notions of what a wheelchair means, that is, not having the ability to walk.[4] Had she been older, such an act may not have been as subversive because it is more common for older people to use wheelchairs or scooters to maneuver shopping malls and city streets. Or had she been among friends at home, the impact would not have been the same. Her act is destabilizing because there are no competing scripts writing her body as potentially disabling and the audience has no prior knowledge of her illness.

Visibility of chronic illness and disability resulting from RA contrasts sharply with that of ME. The common complaint that no one "sees" ME—something that is important socially because such women with ME "look" okay and seem to be healthy. Knowledge about ME is invisible to mainstream society and not well known to the general public and, in addition, is sometimes dismissed by health practitioners. With many of its dimensions existing in the realm of the unknown, ME is questioned because there is no known permanent damage to the body; there is no known cause of illness; there is no known successful treatment. Even though the course of ME is unpredictable, fluctuating, and individual, just like many other more "legitimate" chronic illnesses that have obtained the stamp of medical authority, this imprecise pattern is used against women with symptoms associated with ME. Because of the difficulties in the way ME as a disease manifests in the body, many physicians indicate that the illness is unreal and suggest the cause of the fluctuation is actually a psychological or psychiatric disorder, a manifestation of stress, or something else "in your head."[5] Raquel noted this type of invisibility, and tried to explain it in terms of a bodily, material, concrete struggle.

It's like I can feel the cells in my body sort of battle. It's really hard to describe, but I, it's like I'm aware that my whole system is constantly fighting something. . . . When you stabilize your, what they measure every month is my para-protein level. Abnormal protein level. And I stabilized it so that on a scale of one to thirty, once you get past ten, you start getting twitches. Mine's been stabilized at seven, but my immune system is at three. And your immune system, I think is supposed to be around ten or fifteen. Better at fifteen from what I understand. So I have a very low immune system which is normal for somebody who'd got this para-protein problem. But that means I always feel like I've got the flu. And my body is always fighting. And so when I sleep, I am mostly aware of it in the afternoon when I sleep. It's just very interesting. And it's quite, I just feel everything moving. And everything is kind of agitated. And I can see it. Just literally see it, like there is this war going on. It's very difficult to describe. And at times, like I say, I almost feel like I am observing this process. And I think that when I sleep, because I need to sleep, because that's the time when this battle actually happens, it makes it so that I am okay. It's really strange. Very strange.

Raquel's metaphor of her body as a battlefield is consistent with many of the discourses invoked to describe illness.[6] The physical sensations of the battle remain invisible and highly suspect by the physicians she has seen because her description does not "fit" what it is to be ill. Yet she talks about her body in medical terms; she seems to have intricate knowledge about the relationship between her immune system and para-protein levels and is reading her body through test results; it is this biomedical knowledge through which she is interpreting what is happening in and to her body. But Raquel could easily have been speaking figuratively about the discursive inscription of ME onto a body with chronic pain, chronic infection, and chronic fatigue. Over a period of fourteen years, Raquel was variously diagnosed with Myelodysplasia Syndrome and Fibromyalgia Syndrome, and, in the biomedical search for the genesis of pain, surgeons removed her thyroid gland and both ovaries. Interactions between heavy drugs and her body, as well as the various surgical procedures, set her body up as both a figurative and a literal battleground. On the battleground of her body, physicians sought to figure out what was *wrong* with her—labeling her, then operating; constructing a discourse of deviance, then using material interventions—all in an attempt to make visible, in some way, the constellation of symptoms eventually designated as ME.

ILLNESS AND ENVIRONMENT

The discursive inscriptions of chronic illness and disability are part of the constitution of the experience of the physical sensations of the body, women's embodiment. Also part of this constitution is the physical environment within which the women live their daily lives, women's corporeal space. Compounding the limiting of the material body due to the disease process is a sense of confinement through being tied to a particular place. Arranging daily living activities around the physical sensations of pain and fatigue and the uncertainty of bodily functioning sometimes restricts women with chronic illness to familiar places, such as homes and their beds, bathrooms, and stairs. Throughout Gwen's account of her experiences of chronic illness, she refers to "lack of control"—physically, financially, and emotionally. Gwen counters this destabilization by asserting control over her physical environment.

> Well, it's just you haven't got the freedom of traveling, doing things like that. There is no way I want to travel and wake up in a bed where I am in the "sag" and I am in a strange bed in a strange town. I couldn't do it. These are the kinds of things that bother me. But then, I've got a nice place to live now so I am not too worried. I mean if I were coming in like a lot of the women I know, they've got one bedroom, a little sitting room and that's it. Well, you know, I think I would go a little stir crazy in that. Because I go around and around.

Loss of freedom to do everyday things, which may be something as simple as walking around the garden, contribute to the constitution of the experience of being ill and having an ill body. Although for the most part invisible, such a border enhances the possibilities women with chronic illness have to negotiate the physical limits of their bodies. At the same time, that same border complicates women's abilities to attend to a body with uncertain and fluctuating symptoms. For example, socializing helps in lessening the extreme isolation women feel when ill. Yet venturing out of comfortable surroundings can cause anxiety over the ability to control a "chaotic" body. Because of the instability of the women's bodies, this border, too is unstable—sometimes being "closer in," sometimes "further away," creating a situation where social engagements are sometimes kept and sometimes broken.

What constitutes the flexibility in these material borders—of the body and of the living environment—is the variability of dominance in symptoms. The nature of chronicity involves an ongoing ebb and flow of not only the intensity of a particular sensation, but also the configuration of sensations. As Gwen's experiences have already demonstrated, control over the physical aspects of a woman's home environment can create a relatively comfortable living space. This control over one's immediate surroundings is not always possible. Janet, an athlete who trained regularly, experienced a sudden onset of RA. Although she had severe pain, she did not have fatigue, so she continued working at the small home service company without even trying to adjust her work schedule. Eventually the company dissolved and Janet moved to freelance work. Even though this was not a planned change, Janet likes freelancing because she is able to adjust her work according to her bodily limits within her home space. For Rhonda, fatigue has developed as her most problematic symptom. At onset, she was just finishing university and was able to create a research position for herself. With the assistance of her previous employer, she moved into consulting work soon thereafter. She has much control over her work environment, now located in her home space, which supports her negotiation of fatigue on a daily basis.

Together these examples show how the corporeality of chronic illness is filtered through women's embodiment. Discursive and material bodies manifested through inscription are synchronous. As women engage the environments around them, they continually negotiate the material limits of their bodies in the context of the immediacy of their surroundings. The palpability of illness exudes beyond the body into the environment as that space becomes livable or limiting for women with chronic illness. The materiality of these spaces both enables women to live relatively comfortably and closes off access to other environments, as for example, friends' homes, restaurants, or new workplaces. In this latter sense, the materiality of the environment limits the body. Yet these borders emerge as flexible, permeable, negotiable boundaries. They are fixed only temporarily at a specific time, in a particular space, thus providing room for women to accommodate their "chaotic" bodies. Engaging these borders influences the constitutive processes of their bodies and texture their corporeal space.

ADJUSTMENT TO DAILY ROUTINES

The strategies by which women accommodate their "chaotic" bodies vary. The women diagnosed with ME talked more about the physicality of their illness in terms of the arrangement of their daily activities than the women with RA. Women with RA tended to focus on detailing specific tasks. We think that this is probably the case because of the intensity of fatigue experienced by women with ME, where combing hair, brushing teeth, or another mundane task may be overwhelming and cause for an afternoon's rest.

For women with RA, avoiding tasks that cause pain are a priority. For example, Sara described putting on face cream.

> I don't have any strength in my hands. These two fingers have locked in the bent position. And I think that's because of the nerve here. And they are a bit numb. And this of course, the last joint is bent. And so with this left hand, my thumb isn't good. But in this hand, my middle finger is the only one, if I put cream on my face, that's the only finger I can use. And then I have to support my hand too. I don't have the strength, I have to support it, and that helps. Now I can't use my right hand to put cream on my face, or whatever, because it's curved and if I did, the nails would dig in my face. You know what I mean? So you learn that you can't do this and you can't do that. So you have to devise ways and means of getting around those situations.

This tactile sketch of face cream application demonstrates the way in which women use their experience as a basis to make decisions about activities to accommodate their bodily limits. Applying face cream is a seemingly trifling, mundane task, but it is through the destabilization of these types of tasks that women with chronic illness are able to reconfigure what is common sense. Redefining common sense contributes to the contestation of normalizing and naturalizing processes that shape discursive and material bodies. Accessing common sense in order to challenge the specificity of a women's embodiment may also entail tasks associated with maintaining a home or being part of a family. When accommodating illness or an ill body, women may choose to let the dishes pile up higher, the floors get dirtier, and grass grow longer. They may also choose to see close friends only, go out less often, and plan to attend social events sparingly.

Arranging everyday life around bodily limits often means spacing tasks out over an entire day. A typical day for Connie, for example, revolves around caring for her ill body while at the same time meeting her familial obligation of preparing supper. Once getting out of bed at about seven in the morning:

> I come in the living room and have my coffee and a couple of cigarettes, read the paper. And then I let the dog in. . . . And then I watch 2 soap operas. . . . But I tape yesterday's and then I watch them in the morning so that I can fast forward through the commercials and also through the really boring parts. And then I usually read, because I've watched my soap operas, and I take all my medication. And I usually lay on the sofa and read or go to bed and read and sleep. Now it depends on the night's sleep. If I've had a good night's sleep I don't go to bed until 1:00, when I sleep for an hour and a half. If I've had a disturbed night's sleep I will sleep in the morning for an hour and a half and again in the afternoon from about 2:00 to 4:00. I give myself that time for quietness and if I nod off that's fine and if I don't that's okay too. I just stay really quiet.

The rest of her day is much the same. During the later afternoon she'll slowly make supper, peeling potatoes or snap green beans at her leisure. During supper, it is too noisy, so she usually eats by herself. The evening is full of more rest, but mostly in the bedroom. Sometimes her two teenaged daughters visit or they watch TV together. At nine o'clock her husband comes to bed and watches TV for an hour or so. Then she sleeps again until around midnight, when she'll write or rest or read until three or four in the morning. And then fall sleep until the next day starts at seven.

Connie's day is like the days of many of the women with ME. Resting, reading, watching television, minimal interaction, and "saving" your energy for something special. In contrast, Helen, diagnosed with RA, organizes her day quite differently, but with a similar set of principles—"saving" energy during some parts of the day so that you can expend it when you need it.

> Although I am not working [in paid labor], my work day basically begins at four [in the afternoon], whereas everybody else who doesn't have kids goes to work at nine o'clock and makes it home by four. And if you've got RA and you've managed to struggle through that whole day, [so] at four o'clock you can walk in the door and go right to bed and not cook dinner or anything else. At four, my day begins . . . I then have to stay up for the evening. I make dinner. I supervise housework. I supervise homework. I have to be cheerful. I have to be nice to my husband. You know, that's my work day.

This arrangement works well for Helen—she is able to exert herself when necessary within her own home environment, while still being part of the family. Setting up a routine can be comforting for women with chronic illness because they may be more readily able to negotiate the borders of illness within a set of temporal parameters. However, this balance between rest and work, as Helen shows, is delicate.

Well, on weekends, all of a sudden, I go from . . . 8:30 in the morning until after ten at night. Ten at night during the week may be okay to go to bed early and everybody else is going to bed early. But it's very hard when everybody's watching a movie at 11:00 and you go to bed. When by 11:00 it's exhausting and you're ready for bed, but your husband's energy level has just gotten up. And you know? So weekends, I do find difficult, especially. I think it's hard, especially in the summer and things.

When actively engaging the flexibility of these borders that Helen describes, women create elaborate routines in order to be able do what it is they want to do. Margie's experiences show how the organization of her time and space permit her to work part-time as a receptionist. She lives alone and receives home support, funded through the state.

I use up a lot of energy just getting up in the morning and getting dressed, making myself a cup of tea and showering and, I—you know, I get dressed, most of my clothes on, and then the homemaker comes about ten o'clock. She does my shoes and socks and she'll help me with my hair a bit, and make me some breakfast, and [then] I get ready for work. And I leave for work and I'm there all afternoon. Come home and have dinner, and I usually don't go out on weeknights, but with the [housing] co-op there's things I have to get involved in here, and there's usually maybe two meetings a month that I have to go to. . . . For a while I was on the board, like, the Board of Directors, and that was really involved, that was a big, really, too involved. So through the week it's pretty quiet, you know. Except on my day off, which is Wednesday, I use that as my day to go out, either to a doctor's appointment or shopping or whatever I need to get out, you know, at a store or whatever.

Margie organizes her home environment to sustain her employment. She could spend more time socializing in the evenings and resting during the day, or more time involved with her housing co-op instead of working out-side the home, but she chooses to remain employed. Being able to exert this type of control over her home environment permits Margie to reconfigure the limits *of* her material body in a way that opens up opportunities once closed to women like her using wheelchairs and *to* her material body so that her lived space include places "beyond these four walls."[7]

Contrasting the lived spaces of Connie, Helen, and Margie provides insight into the significance of adjusting daily routines to accommodate a destabilized/destabilizing body. Chronic illness filters the way in which they live their spaces. Connie is confined to her house, and in fact rarely ventures beyond three rooms—the living room, the kitchen, and the bedroom—unless she has a health-related appointment. Helen, although for the most part confined to the house, is able to roam around the entire house, but is restricted during flare-ups to be within a half an hour's drive of a rheumatologist. Margie, even though she is confined to her home, workplace, and nearby shops, has the most mobility and her lived space encompasses the most territory. Connie's bodily limitations are supposedly reversible in that ME apparently does not cause permanent damage to the material body. Helen's and Margie's limitations are fixed and "permanent" in the sense that the damage to the body by the physiological processes of the disease cannot be reversed; the damage can only be repaired.

We have been able to pull out from these experiences of women with chronic illness one specific strategy that they use to accommodate their "chaotic" bodies, that of adjusting daily routines. Whether inscriptions are discursive—Sandra is concerned about her attractiveness because of a weight gain—or material—Carolyn needs supervision while sleeping so as not to stop breathing—women's bodies are continually in a state of flux with their borders shrinking and expanding unpredictably. Yet, within this chaos, by focusing attention on bodily limits at this fine scale, we are able to indicate at least in a small way how women come to exist within and negotiate these borders constitutive of their corporeal space. They hold in tension the specificity of their bodies at any given moment in any particular place.

SECURING INCOME

Much of the research around women, work, and chronic illness has shown that women are marginalized in employment in a number of ways—in hiring, through accommodation strategies, with little or no benefits, threatened job security, and lower pay.[8] These works, while attending to the links between the characteristics of a specific chronic illness and the limitations it places on a woman in the workplace, try to account for the social and economic context of employment at the same time. It has been a long-standing substantiated contention that women with disabilities are indeed underrepresented in the labor force, receive lower wages, and have fewer job opportunities than either able-bodied women or men with disabilities.[9] In addition to being marginalized as women and as persons with disabilities, women with disabilities who are engaged in both paid employment and maintaining a household face further problems.[10] It is likely that women with chronic illness will have only minimal assistance in the home or in care facilities, unless they have daughters.[11] These arrangements are not only gendered but also racialized.[12] Women receiving such assistance and/or care will also likely have contradictory experiences of receiving care, particularly because they have been "socialized" to be carers.[13] Increasing in the literature are narratives of chronic illness that emphasize the complex entwinements of caregiving, care receiving, and employment. With growing attention on experience in the cultural turn in health sciences, research often includes what has come to be referred to as "the patient's perspective."[14] Taking into account the experience of those with chronic illness is slowly transforming the way in which health and illness are defined, policy is written, and health services delivered—all of which affect women's material circumstances of everyday life.

For the women who already have chronic illness, this change toward including experience of chronic illness, although desirable, is not dealing with the immediate concerns of women who already have chronic illness, that is, of securing income from employers, insurance companies, and the state. The women we talked with struggled over securing some financial support through employment or disability pension. For example, Angel worked for a marketing firm at the onset of RA. She collected information in person, at various homes across the city, traveling on foot, during a time when her feet were swollen and painful. She knew that if she revealed her illness to her employer, she would be fired because she could not do the job. Eventually, she moved to an office and sought advice from a company doctor. In her discussion of her illness with the doctor—something that would definitely be revealed to her employer—she was able to claim that she could complete all the tasks associated with her job description for she no longer was required to walk the streets. The income was important for she was solely responsible for the money needed to raise her two children.

Not all women are able to approach employment and illness the same way Angel did—put off revelation of illness until it is advantageous to do so. Disclosure is a tricky process. By not disclosing illness, women suffer pain, fatigue, and embarrassment while struggling with the limits of their material bodies to undertake their specific tasks. They exist in a state of fear of being "found out," defined as a failure, and reproached for being inadequate. Job security is threatened. Women may go to great lengths to keep their illness invisible to their employers for fear of losing their job. By disclosing illness in the workplace, women's bodies are open to scrutiny. Because chronic illness fluctuates so unpredictably, this surveillance acts as a constant reminder that illness needs to be made visible, for without visibility, there is no "evidence," no proof that illness exists. Omnipresence of the need to demonstrate illness threatens to inscribe women with chronic illness as inadequate and failures, and may jeopardize job security.

This possibility of the intensity of this scrutiny compelled Julia to "hide" her illness from everyone but her (sympathetic) boss and to normalize her public behavior.[15] By developing ways to work "smarter," by expending less energy and being in a position to hire an assistant, Julia was successful in refusing to disclose that she was ill or had been diagnosed with ME. Yet for many other women, disclosure resulted in forms of support. For Sandra, who worked in a medical clinic, disclosure meant that a physician could monitor the progress of the disease and that coworkers could discretely step in and take over her tasks when necessary. Many of the women found supportive environments where disclosure facilitated the possibility of continued employment rather than complicating employment matters: Alex's boss arranged for office equipment to be set up in Alex's home; Gina created her own part-time job; Verna, Rhonda, and Janet pursued freelance work; and Janice negotiated a part-time teaching position. Other women were able to structure their work environment to accommodate the limits to their material body. Initially, Elise cut back her private counseling practice while remaining employed so as to keep her benefits package. When her employer added a wing onto the building, Elise moved there because of the toxicity of her previous office locations—near chlorine fumes. Once it became clear that the carpet in the new building was a problem, her employer arranged to solve the problem. Pauline's and Brie's employers offered a range of options for maintaining employment; however, neither could remain employed.

These experiences of supportive work environments that have been restructured to accommodate the destabilized/destabilizing body do not coincide with the fear most of the same women expressed of losing their job. We don't think that this is because the threat of job loss is not there, it is; rather, it is because the threat itself of losing the job figures prominently in the notion of work.[16] Discourses reinforcing the notion of a healthy, working body coupled with those sustaining the precariousness of any employment in an era of restructuring and downsizing, obliges women to naturalize the idea that to be a good worker is to have control of their bodies. For women with "chaotic," destabilizing bodies, prior to diagnosis, it would be difficult to identify a "legitimate" reason for not being able to work. For example, Dolores and Teresa both suffered from severe back pain that was exacerbated by the work they did in hospital. Although both were eventually diagnosed with ME, Dolores was able to secure long-term disability benefits prior to being diagnosed, but Teresa was not. Dolores was able to demonstrate with "evidence" from physicians that she was not able to be a "good worker" for *legitimate* reasons—her back injury, received on the job, precluded her from performing all her duties. In contrast, Teresa was not able to trace her pain to a particular injury at a specific point in time and thus was not able to be a "good worker," period. She was only able to say that she was in pain. So, instead of pursuing a quest for a diagnosis in hopes of *legitimating* her bodily sensations, she quit, thereby losing access to all benefits. A few years later, she was diagnosed with Fibromyalgia Syndrome and ME.

Definitions of being ill are continually negotiated in the workplace. For example, even though Eve had a (moral and legislative) right to take time off at the onset of RA, she was reticent to use her "sick days" because she was afraid she might get "sick"! The invisibility of RA in the context of her definition of illness—presumably acute, life-threatening illness—filtered her response to her own embodiment of chronic illness. When Reann approached her employer to discuss taking sick leave, the interaction demonstrates that the immediacy of the chronicity of illness is not usually visible: "I told him that I was not doing well and I couldn't continue work. And he asked me 'well, when do you want to leave?' And he opened up his calendar, you know, hoping he could see down the road. And I said, 'Today.' I said, 'Today—I've got to leave today.'" After some time away from the workplace, Reann returned part-time.

> I . . . found that after the first month I came back, when I was working part-time, that it kind of worked its way back into full-time, because they kept on asking me to do stuff. And then I stopped and looked and, oh, I'm back at full time again. You know? And it was always pressure. Being pressured to do extra work. And it was like a 24-hour call service. It was wild and even though I asked to be totally removed from that, it didn't work out that way. So, I don't know. And there are certain jobs that, I don't know. You almost have to re-design the job. Because there are some things in a job that you can't expect to go back to. You know, like mopping floors, pushing a thirty-pound mop around the floor when you have Fibromyalgia. That doesn't work. Actually, it's quite painful.

For Reann, re-entry into the workplace, even a reduced workload, did not signal any change in working habits. Within the month she was back to all her tasks, full-time.[17] In a workplace context, it is difficult to maintain an in-between state of being where a worker can be sick, but engaging in paid work.[18] The ability to do this will also be conditioned by the type of workplace, with fast-paced performance-based private companies being less tolerant than some public corporations, and where a woman's track record on the job or highly specialized skills are valued.

Defining what constitutes illness in the workplace is also negotiated outside the workplace in institutions that make decisions about possible income for women with chronic illness—state bureaucracies administering disability pension plans and private insurance companies administering long-term disability policies. Margrit Shildrick and Janet Price show how forms for state-sponsored funding for disability benefits set strict parameters for defining the disabled body.[19] Their observations could easily be applied to private insurance disability claim forms. Two relevant points arise from their work with regard to our interpretation here. First, persons with chronic illness, although disabled in the sense of not being able to perform the tasks that they could prior to onset of illness, are not always deemed disabled when appealing to these policies. The policy language, even in its own ambiguity, arranges the scrutiny of the applicant's body to be self-revealing, as for example, the detailed questions about toilet needs in terms of time spent on toilet needs, tasks needing attention, and competency in being able to perform the tasks. This line of questioning does not take into account the *need* to be near a bathroom around the clock, the inaccessibility of toilets in public places, or the fluctuation in toilet needs for women with chronic illness; it only includes the tasks associated with toilet needs—urination, menstrual flow, and bowel movements. This self-surveillance replaces the state's gaze but still focuses disability on individual failing rather than social or environmental factors. Instead of scrutinizing women's corporeal space, state policies designating disability fragment all bodies into individual tasks and body parts— closely measuring their inadequacy. For women with chronic illness, this self-surveillance is often askew to what is taxing a woman's body—the way the body parts work together. For example, at one point in time a woman with ME may be able to walk a city block, perhaps two. But the "disability" comes afterwards when exhaustion hits and the woman must lie down for several hours afterwards—a question that covers the immediacy and urgency of the rest does not exist on the form.[20] Or a woman can do some parts of her job, like typing, but cannot consistently remember the codes for data entry. If there is room on the forms for this type of self-scrutiny, claims have to be corroborated by tests conducted by physicians, such a serial sevens, walking a line heel-toe, and an upright tilt-table test.[21] This corroboration is necessary if a woman wants to be officially designated as disabled, and her claims of inadequacy taken seriously.

Second, this designation of inadequacy sets the stage for interpreting any claim for disability based on chronic illness as easy to turn down; although ill, an individual may not be able, by the parameters set out in disability insurance applications (which also vary), to be designated as disabled. For chronic illness that has a contestable or no clear diagnosis, like ME, this denial is like being denied, yet again, having the experience of a fatigued, cognitively impaired, pain-infused, ill body invalidated. Many of the women with ME gave details about their struggles with their claims for private and state-sponsored disability benefits. One of the most common themes was denial on biomedical grounds. It is a common belief that ME does not exist as a physical disease, both popularly and among physicians, and is the same as clinical depression. Depression is now considered treatable through either prescription or non-prescription drugs and is not justifiably a long-term disabling chronic illness. What is significant here is that illness, as a discursive category, moves outside the realm of experience and medicine into the realm of allocating incomes for persons with disabilities. With this discursive move, the institutions distributing money redefine *materially* what it is to be ill. For example, Sophie was experiencing symptoms associated with ME intense enough to prevent her from working as a medical technologist, and went to her physician to seek treatment. He diagnosed depression and prescribed a pharmaceutical and more exercise. She did not improve. Struggles ensued between herself (trying to convince her physician she was not depressed and that there was something physiologically [material] going on with her body) and her physician (who did not "believe in" ME and was empirically sorting her symptoms into the discursive category of depression) and the insurance company, who appropriated the discursive category of depression and set parameters for being ill (depression is a legitimate illness whereas ME is not) and determining justifiable treatment (drugs and exercise).[22] She was ordered back to work by the insurance company, and promptly collapsed—three different times after three different attempts to return to work. Her physician finally acknowledged ME and the insurance company was finally convinced of her physical fatigue, cognitive impairment, and ongoing pain.

Another woman's experiences with private and state-sponsored insurance companies—denying her claims initially, then granting the claims after having appealed, and then having to sustain her income by doing what the insurance companies tell her to do—reinforced her ideas about how to use self-surveillance to her advantage.[23] This woman was ill for many years before ME was finally diagnosed.

> And I think it's so important that, it has done good to recognize that the doctors really don't know what. They don't have all the answers. I hate to say this, but I played the game in order to get long-term disability. And I hate it. It absolutely appalls me that that's what you have to do. But it is a game. I go to a psychiatrist every week because I have to show that I cannot go back to work. You know? And also my [doctor], I say "Yes, I will try these things." And I do try them. I mean I am quite honest about it. I tried this medicine and I don't want to take it . . . [words on tape unclear] body because I know my body reacts to it. So it's an interesting factor. If you actually look at the reality of it, it doesn't make sense. And it isn't the right thing to be doing. I mean the system is set up that you haven't a choice. You are without choices if you have to rely on long-term disability. If you are independently wealthy, that's a whole other story. You can do what you want to do. And I know there is a lot of people who needed the work and [words on tape unclear]. . . . It is a reality. I don't think it's fair.

Once the claims were filed and the appeals successful, this woman saw that the only way to keep the discursive category that best describes her experience of chronic illness is to do exactly what she is told. In doing so, she is able to secure an income so that she can concentrate on her healing.

What these examples show is that securing financial support is linked to the materiality of chronic illness and its discursive construction. Discursive categories of material bodies as well as the material bodies themselves participate in constituting chronic illness *as* chronic illness. Details of the experience of this constitution are substantially shaped by the material conditions within which women with chronic illness live. Economically, the most vulnerable were those women not employed at the time of onset. Debby and Yvonne were students at the onset of ME. Debby collapsed during term and did not complete her studies. She was living on her own and soon after getting ill moved in with her mother, with whom she has lived for the ten years she has been ill. Debby is completely dependent financially on her mother, as is Yvonne on her father. Because of the breakdown of the immune system of her body, Yvonne needed to live in a chemical-free environment. Her father rents and paid for limited renovations of a house out in the country. Her father gives her a living allowance and pays for her psychotherapy sessions.

Belle and Carolyn have always had income from provincial disability grants. Belle lives with her parents in her own living space and contributes to household maintenance—much like a roommate arrangement. She also does some tutoring of school-aged children. Carolyn lives on her own and accesses subsidized home care services. Leeza, Fern, Stella, and Shelagh do not derive any income from disability insurance, although Shelagh is appealing her denial of a state pension. All are financially dependent on their husbands, or ex-husband in Stella's case, and have limited or no access to the relatively low incomes their husbands earn. Barbara, too, is financially dependent on her husband who, however, earns a substantial income. She was employed at the time of onset of RA, and quit because of the problems she was having with fatigue and pain. Her husband supported her throughout this period and continues to do so.

The unevenness in financial support for women with chronic illness by individuals and by institutions matters in the approach to dealing with the treatment for chronic illness. Some women, like Renee, have difficulties scraping together enough money for bus fare to go to a support group meeting, whereas Elise had the money to re-do her entire house to accommodate her sensitivities. Barbara has the money to hire a nanny to assist her in raising her three children whereas Gina is unable to assist her children in even the simplest of tasks. Many of the women choose to treat their illness with alternative or complementary medicine, including for example traditional Chinese medicine, homeopathy, naturopathy, psychotherapy, food supplements, and hydro-, physio-, and massage therapy. Most medical plans do not cover the entire cost of these treatments, if they cover any cost at all. So only the women who can afford it undertake these treatments. Many of the low-income women expressed how much they would like to try alternative therapies, but are not able to because of the cost.

FLUID, PERMEABLE LIMITS

Fluidity and permeability of borders is a common theme in poststructural accounts of identities and bodies.[24] Within the narratives of these women with chronic illness, there was a theme that once bodily limits are recognized, coping with chronic illness can begin. The recognition of a seemingly "fixed" location of a border acts as a moment of epiphany wherein the women experience the limit of their material bodies, as exemplified by Dolores' comment, "And I used to be so tired that I could never feel that and it was just such an improvement when I could actually feel that and know I was that tired. That was a big turn around in my limits. To recognize it. To acknowledge it." Rather than conceptualizing a limit as either a constraint or as an impervious boundary, we think that this "turn-around" Dolores speaks of is actually the recognition of the permeability and fluidity of a limit. For women with chronic illness, these material limits come into focus because of the destabilization of the material body in sensations of pain, fatigue, and cognitive impairment, and the discursive one, in categories that are ascribed then taken away and reascribed.

Throughout this chapter we have shown how the materiality of illness, in terms of both physiology and economy, is constitutive of the bodily limits these women experience. Through careful action with adequate resources, women can negotiate their social and physical environments to accommodate their chronic illness. For us, this means that women with chronic illness come to embody these limits—constitutive of both their materiality and discourse—as a way to redefine the parameters within which they exist as "bodies in context." Our account of the women's experience show how their embodiment in the corporeal spaces of home and workplace environments constitute these borders as permeable and fluid, drawing directly from their experiences of their own fluctuating bodies with chronic illness.

8

Absence of Presence/Presence of Absence: Borders, Identity, Everyday Life

I need a nap. Right now. I just have to make it home. These errands. It wouldn't be fair to dump them on Danielle, or would it? She might like to drive. Just one more thing. The post office. I'll be done and then I get to lie down. My bed. My pillow. . . . I hope Mom likes these candlesticks. I could take them to her. But not until the week after next, after her birthday. That wouldn't be okay. This weekend is Ladysmith. Right. That's right. The week after next. Maybe I'll go see Jenny, too. But the trip is so long. I better not tell them that I'm thinking of coming. They'll just end up expecting me. And when I don't show up. . . . I don't want to have to explain. They don't need to know, not everything at least. They would just worry. I don't want them thinking that I can't do everything myself. . . . It's so different now. I can't do anything. And there's so much to do. I've got to see Mom and Jenny, live with Danielle, teach all those kids. Sometimes it's just too much. . . . Where did I go? Change. Maybe that's what I need. But who do I want to be? . . . "Yes, and a book of stamps. That's all." . . . My keys? Where are my keys? . . . Okay, here they are. I'm done. I get to lie down. . . . Oh yeah. That construction. Which way do I go? Stop. Just take your time. Think. . . . I don't. I can't. I must be losing my mind. I can't remember anything. . . . Oh yeah, that's right. I've got to go right. . . . What am I thinking? I'm not going to be able to go anywhere. Why do I do this to myself? I'll have to phone Ross and tell him I can't go. He won't understand. He never does. . . . Right. Don't even think about going.

Identities of women with chronic illness fluctuate, vary in time across space, and are temporarily "fixed." They emerge in relation to "bodies in

125

context" and are fragile in expression, constituted through a woman's specific embeddedness within complex webs of social relations and particular(ized) deployments of power. Women with chronic illness come to know themselves and come to express who they are as mothers, employees, wives, partners, daughters, and women *with chronic illness* through the mediation of specific configurations of power/knowledge/space. Yet any identity, contingent in its articulation, is unstable, ready to be de-linked and re-linked to a different set of relations or in a different space. The instability of any one identity is heightened for women with chronic illness because of the state of flux their bodies are in. Such unpredictable movement promotes a sense of chaos, something that women struggling with symptoms of pain, fatigue, loss of fine motor skills, or other physical symptoms find disconcerting.

These fluctuating identities are not completely formed, nor monolithic. Because of the process of identity formation through the "constitutive outside," any manifest identity carries with it parts of identities that have been denied and excluded, such as a healthy person not being chronically or acutely ill and vice versa. For women with chronic illness, the negotiation of such matters in producing and reproducing a notion of self is jumbled up—at some moments, health dominates; at others, illness; and at still others, health and illness exist without the need to claim or reject either. Because women with chronic illness embody the muddled borders of health and illness, their embeddedness within specific deployments of power/knowledge/space influences how, when, and where a particular identity manifests, or following Chantal Mouffe's arguments, how, when, and where a nodal point emerges around which an identity can coalesce.[1] Multiple discourses involving women, their definition, and the setting of parameters for their actions inscribe the bodies of women with chronic illness with contradictions that the women themselves have to mediate, both as individuals and as "bodies in context."

The course charted here supports the notion that identities are transitory, moving from one to another and then to another depending on the contingencies of context. For women with chronic illness, these transitory identities are results of their immediate and long-term negotiations of power through their own embodiment. In conceiving the body as both a site of oppression and a site of resistance *at the same time*, we are able to indicate ways through which women mediate power and negotiate self. Although women are marginalized in social, financial, and medical contexts, they are able to resist complete dominance of hegemonic discourses and social practices that define the women's ill bodies and that set parameters for women's behavior. We have shown in previous chapters how discursive notions of women with chronic illness affect experiences of illness and health and how the materiality of the body and the conditions within which women live constrain the choices women have to accommodate their bodies physically and socially.

We have also shown how these notions and conditions limit the body and how women resist bodily restrictions. Within this milieu, the mediation of power continually takes place as women make sense of their synchronous experience of bodily sensations and bodily meanings. As constellations of symptoms shift, as diagnoses change, as finances become unstable so too do demands on time and energy, expectations of tasks, and images of achievement. While the immediacy of responding to change for women with chronic illness languishes into flexible patterns of self over weeks, months, and years, the process of mediation is ongoing, albeit in fits and starts.

Sorting through the processes of self formation and those through which women come to a particular(ized) identity involves the linking and de-linking of self and identity within a specific configuration of social relations and their specificity, expressed through power/knowledge/space. In mediating various articulations of power, women emerge on occasion with a particular-(ized) identity, "fixed" temporarily, creating a *specific* body. For women with chronic illness, this emergence is then eclipsed by another emergent identity, mediated through the same power relations but has been, at least momentarily, differently articulated, creating yet another *specific* body. Although the deployment of power plays a significant role in defining any configuration of social relations, women are not subject to complete dominance of a singular conception of illness. Within any power/knowledge/space regime, there is space for negotiation and resistance. That identities—individual and collective—can be conceived as transitory for women with chronic illness means that we can access (conceptually and concretely) how women maneuver through constitutive processes of self and find expressions of their own fleeting, contradictory, and transitory identity(ies). Through this negotiation of meaning and matter, women engage in a process of re-cognition—re-learning their body vis-à-vis self. Depending in part on the concreteness of the disease process and in part on other aspects of women's experiences of chronic illness, the space for re-cognition available to women is variously constrained. Just as the women are embedded within the social relations of power/knowledge/space and circumscribed by bodily discourses and materialities, so too are their efforts to resist.

One way to contribute to understanding experiences of women with chronic illness is to scrutinize the process through which women come to an understanding of self as they negotiate their identities through their own embodiment. If, as we claim, identities are fluctuating and transitory, what becomes an issue is how to gain access to a temporally and spatially "fixed" identity without naturalizing any one identity. In the rest of this chapter, we illustrate these points by concentrating on the women's experiences of their transitions from relative health to chronic illness in relation to formation of self and expression of identity. We first describe a prominent theme surfacing in the women's stories, that of a focus on the absence of a presence and the presence of absence. We then elaborate our arguments about embodying borders set out at the end of the previous chapter and look in detail, through two examples, at how women may seek out a space to be ill. We next turn to showing how some women move toward a "new" self, often phrased in terms of grieving losses and to drawing attention to how women reconstitute their identities *with* illness. As an extension, we explore how this presence of absence manifests through choices women make about disclosing their illness to family, friends, coworkers, and employers alongside some of the possible repercussions. Finally, we move toward opening up a discussion about expressions of identity in the everyday spaces women with chronic illness traverse.

ABSENCE AND PRESENCE

Onset of illness brings into focus the social and physical milieu through which issues about self and identity surface. Through depictions of shifts in relationships, the women conveyed the meaning of their transition from health to illness as one of uncertainty. Many of the women set up their stories of the onset of illness in the context of family and friends. Jayne, for example, discussed her role as mother to two teenagers, continuing into the first two years of her illness.

> Well with my children, they were with me when I got sick. They were 19 or 20, I guess, or 18 or 19 and my son had graduated and he was working in retail. He was partying, you know things that 19-year-olds do and I found it very difficult. And he found it difficult because he was used to me being this "super mom." And here I was in bed most of the time and not able to make myself feel better, let alone him [feel better]. He was angry. So that was difficult. And finally after about I guess ten months, almost a year, I asked him if he would leave home until I got better. And that was difficult but he saw how upset I was in having to make that decision, and he left, and now it's great. It took about three or four months after that for him to get over his own feelings of being rejected by it [request for him to leave]. . . . And now he's great. He's still a 21-year-old, you know, involved in his own life and he comes around once a week, sometimes more . . . but it's nice now. . . . My daughter stayed home until she graduated and she made arrangements to live with a friend in an apartment. She was ready to fly. Always ready to fly. And it's been quite wonderful for her because she's [now] got her apartment, she lives on her own, she cooks, cleans, and she phones every day. She comes over once a week. . . . When I had a bad relapse last summer she came and vacuumed and helped me. But I can also see it's difficult for her because she's kind of like I am in that "wanting to be a good girl" stuff. I want to reassure her that it's okay but it's a tricky thing to do because you say, and I know inside, when I had a relapse again, I was so grateful to her for vacuuming. You know that it was

really good. And she said, "It helps me, Mom, because it makes me to not feel as if I've abandoned you." That was the first real clue that I had, you know, all those things that you don't think of people. So I'm glad she's not home in many ways. And in some ways it's freer for me too, because I know she's okay.

Jayne, like many of the women, struggled with her and her children's expectations of being a mother while being ill. Late nights and worrying about her son proved to be "too difficult" for her—both in terms of negotiating motherhood and of dealing with the physical strain on her body. After her son's move, and some time for adjustment, the relationship improved as Jayne re-negotiated expectations of mothering. Jayne's experiences also indicate that she was aware of reproducing and naturalizing, in her relationship with her daughter, a strong caring ethic usually reserved for women. She was torn between not wanting her daughter to be a "good girl," providing unconditional support and care at the drop of the hat, and being grateful that her daughter assisted her when she had a relapse, precluding self care. Through these relationships, Jayne works through her own notion of self and exploring spaces on the borders to bring to bear her "new" identity as a mother who happens to have a chronic illness.

In Jayne's story of her relationships with her children, there is an underlying notion that the "real mother" is absent, having been replaced by an "ill woman," one who needs a lot of attention emotionally so as to be able to sort through who she was before getting ill and who she wants to be after she recovers. Knowing who she is *now*—as a mother, as a woman—is not a priority; the search for meaning is what is at issue. "But also I think that I guess I've learned things about myself, you know, it sounds like a long time to search for meaning, doesn't it? [The two years I've been ill]. . . . I was just reading this article last night about searching for meaning and it was like, 'gosh, that's me!' " This focus on identity prior to onset and intense work on self for the future highlights what we would call an absence of presence— the past and the future are primary concerns and the present is something to live through, full of difficult decisions about renegotiating the boundaries of self and expressions of identity.

There also is the presence of absence—women's stories were full of what they considered to be losses, ranging from the inability to play badminton or garden to the loss of "my life" and "me." Connie's description of her reaction to the onset of ME details the difference in her expectation of being ill and in her sense of being let down once she became ill. "And you know, when I got sick I thought, God, I am so angry at you!" At onset of illness, Connie had recently married, bought a house, and gotten a dog she had wanted for years. She had already recovered from alcoholism and breast cancer and felt that she had finally found a place in her life where she was happy. But becoming ill with ME unsettled her sense of happiness. Throughout

Connie's narrative she conveys the sense that she used to have a wonderful life and that she has grand plans for the future. But there is little discussion of the present, except in details of daily living. She recognized this shift away from happiness and named it as "loss," not a loss of health (which would appear to be a common response among women with chronic illness), but simply a "loss." Connie, even when questioned directly, could not pinpoint what it is she "lost" for she was still married, still owned her home, and still had her dog. We think that Connie was actually referring to an absence of presence, something she recognized as a loss and wanted to grieve.

This theme of absence and presence in the context of self and identity permeated the stories of the women diagnosed with RA and ME. Our main goal in interpreting the emergence of identity in the women's narratives was to work through how the women's identities and their sense of self coalesced around these two points.

BORDERS

At the end of the previous chapter, we argued that women with chronic illness experience the material limits of their body, not as solid, impervious boundaries, but as fluid, permeable borders. Like chronic illness itself, these borders wax and wane, briefly congealing to form limits, then quickly dissolving so as to permit a new border to take shape. In order to contend with this fluctuating pattern of bodily border formation, women with chronic illness forged spaces to negotiate the discursive and material limits of the body. They moved with the uneven expansion and contraction of these borders, taking up the unpredictability of form and shape by *living* these spaces. Through this type of embodiment, they were able to engage in redefining the parameters of what it is to be ill socially and physically as well as of the social and physical environments they come to inhabit. For women with chronic illness, identities and notions of self emerge through embodying limits of the body and negotiating borders of illness. Accounts of their experiences with these limits and borders show how the women's own identities shifted and changed. Two examples are used to show this process in relation to two different contexts, the paid workplace and home space.

Reann, who had been employed as a science technician in a state institution, points out that making space to be ill in the workplace is not an easy task, especially when the illness itself is contested.

> But I think the one thing, if I had anything to wish for, in a way, would be that it [struggle for legitimacy in being ill] wasn't such an upstream battle. It's that if people were just to accept the fact that this thing [ME as an illness] exists, and that we have to alter our lives to live in society, and that there is

that support and allowances, that that would remove so much stress. . . . But trying to fit in, you know, like a round peg into a square hole, it just can't be done. . . . Both psychologically and physically. So they [people with ME] would never go back to the workplace with that kind of stress. The expectations. I think it's the expectation of trying to fit a role that you know you'll never fit again . . . and that's not the way to live with ME. You're just not going to survive very long. One thing I'll mention that I found really startling is that if you have ME, you can't get life insurance.[2]

For Reann, the struggle for legitimacy in being accepted as being ill and unable to work, shapes how she understands her self. If ME were a "legitimate" illness, then there would not be expectations for her to go back to work; it would be clear that she would not be able to take on the tasks that were her responsibility prior to leaving the workplace. At the same time she recognizes that clinging to the notion that she will "never fit again" is not a way of living with ME, even though social practices, such as being denied access to life insurance, reinforce the notion that a person with ME is no longer a "normal" person. As well, the effort not to struggle to "fit in" in the workplace has dire consequences for the material conditions within which this non-legitimacy is lived—without a job, women can only access the minimum benefits available to them through the state.

The workplace is not the only place where women with chronic illness embody limits and borders. Brie's account of her experiences of the shifts she encountered in her notion of self as a woman with chronic illness highlights the instability of any one expression of identity in another context.

I was having a very fine life, I thought. You know, out and about socially, you know. All going pretty well, I thought. Until the abyss [the onset of ME]. So it brought—it questioned everything, in that I was not in control of my life, that there were things that I did not know, could not control. I couldn't get what I wanted, maybe what I wanted was not what I really wanted anyway. And who was it that was wanting it? Was I out there pleasing everyone for my good, because I wanted to? Or because I'd been programmed that way? And the latter is the truth. So it all had to break down.

The catalyst for Brie to embark on a quest for a "new" self was different from Jayne, whose catalyst was negotiating motherhood. Being "out of control" and living in "an abyss" prompted her to re-evaluate her own being in the world. Along with the destabilization of her material body, Brie saw that after the onset of ME it was a good time to "break down" her self, and re-think who she was. Her goal was "to redefine myself as a person, as is. Without any, you know. Whether I'm useless, useful, whatever other terms other people might apply, it doesn't matter now, that I've redefined myself in my own terms. Or else I'm working at that now. Or I am not redefining, I just am. And, you know, something will emerge I suppose."

Brie sought to redefine her self *as is*, through what she refers to as "on her own terms," without the expectations that had shaped her life prior to onset.[3] Yet even in her determined focus on her *being* in context, of her "body in context," she still has an absence of presence—she *supposed* that something, like a self or an identity, would emerge sometime, if not now. She continued, expressing how she was coming to terms with herself and the limits of her body.

> You know, you sort of have one set of symptoms, and they'd shift around, and another set, but you'd still be totally exhausted. You know, so what's that about? I really don't know. I suppose according to what [body part] we've been using more, who knows. . . . I've always done yoga, and so I had a fair amount of mind control and knowledge of meditation. I couldn't do physical things but, you know, I could shut my mind off, stop thinking about that. Shut up, do a mantra, whatever. And that's a great help. You know, and as I say, the drawing, I did a lot of drawing. And the painting, and—used to think I painted a lot, but really, considering the time, I didn't, but I could do so little at a time that it was a focus. And, as I say, it was difficult. You know—so it's still the conflict—you want to do it, you get the stuff out, you do ten minutes, and you know you've had it. Oh well. So I've had it. But I used to fight that. You know. You don't understand why.

Through negotiating the tensions within the borders of the limits of her material body, as for example when she tries to draw but has to put her things away after ten minutes, Brie modifies her understanding of her body. Living the limits of her body means that she does the things that she can actually do, like meditate, draw, or paint, even for a short time—without the expectation that she can do more of any one thing at any one time or do something else entirely at another time. Her reconstituted knowledge of her body involves being who she is at a given point in time, rather than who she used to be, or who she, or someone else, expects her to be.

Brie's account of the process she undertook, and is probably still undertaking, in redefining herself as a person with chronic illness, demonstrates one way a woman with chronic illness lives within the space of her bodily limits—ones that are discursive and material—and negotiates the borders of her illness—discursively and materially. She took on the challenge of engaging the reconstitution of her identity after the destabilization of her material body and actively tried to maneuver through her bodily limits. By becoming aware of the multiple and competing inscriptions on her ill body, she has been sensitized to the discursive as well as the material instability and unpredictability of her body. Holding in tension the borders of her illness, where her body re-forms, she refuses to claim either illness or health; by doing so, she claims both and neither at the same time. Through her bodily activities, she has been able to seek out a space—that has been comforting during her transition—to be whatever it is that *she is* at any given time.

IDENTIFYING AND GRIEVING LOSS

For women with chronic illness, facing illness sometimes shatters the images they have of themselves, somewhat like the process Brie described as a breaking down of both her self and the way she looked at life prior to becoming ill. Entering the transition between being healthy and being chronically ill is perplexing and can be distressing because of the uncertainty in not knowing what the future may be. Will people accept you? Will they understand? Will they reject you? Will you lose your job?

This distress over uncertainty in other people's reactions, about negotiating one's own body in relation to "bodies in context," manifest in the women's stories as a presence of absence—identifying what a woman loses on becoming chronically ill and then dealing with those losses. As Leeza notes, an enormous loss is "your self": "in a way it's like a grieving process. You go through all the emotions of grieving, because your self is gone, and you just have to, yeah, just like losing somebody you love, right?" Entering a transition for women with chronic illness entailed an inventory of losses while at the same time desiring renewal. Even for those few women who found it difficult to remember what it was like at onset of illness, the women recognize that the illness is part of who they are. One of the strategies the women used to recount their experiences of illness is to compare what their life was like prior to onset and what their life was like once ill, with such comparison being more or less explicit

Like Alex, women often listed what it was that they lost upon becoming ill.

> [Y]our loss of your independence, your loss of work, your loss of income, your loss of social life, your loss of help, and you also lose 60% of your income. I spend more on playing around with little medical things than I did on clothes and gas for work. I guess, I'll put it that way. If one of them [disability pensions as an income source] was to be cut off it would be a really, really major problem.

Some losses identified by the women were directly related to the material body and a changed body image. Inge, for example, struggled with her weight gain, both for health reasons—not wanting to be overweight because of her RA—and wanting to be slim so that she would feel attractive. Mary Ann and Sandra were also concerned about being sexually attractive.

Although for some women, like Inge, moving from feeling attractive to engaging in sex encountered other aspects of bodily limits: "making love isn't so much fun—it's kind of like, get this over with, because I've got arthritis." Teresa and Erin both noted that they could no longer lift weights and were thus losing muscle tone. Not being able to exercise was complicating their already complex images of their bodies.

Comparison between what life was like before onset and what life was like after having been ill for some time encompassed more than just body image. Raquel contrasted her former abilities to learn complex tasks with ease to her current difficulty with such learning after having been ill with ME for several years.

> When I first started there [her job] . . . they didn't remember that I was coming on that particular day. And they didn't have a lot for me to do. And so I taught myself with their books and what not and a whole bunch of engineering stuff. . . . And I just learned. I guess that's part of why I get frustrated now is because [of] this dementia now. I know I'm capable of being, even [though my skills are] diminished now. I'm still capable of doing some things. So it's hard, it's really hard. There has been a lot of getting up angry. That part has been difficult and yet I've always said when you lose something, then something else happens to go in a circle. Like the world goes.

Through this comparison, Raquel is able to formulate her cognitive impairment as a presence of absence. Like many of the women in their discussions of losses, Raquel presents at the end of the story an interim solution, something she has come to after grieving with loss. Although difficult, dealing with extreme fuzzy-headedness indicates she is still ill. This resolution is only temporary; she has identified a bodily limit in need of transforming during her state of illness as part of a rejuvenation of self.

Other losses were about being able to engage in some activity, primarily around socializing: traveling, going to the movies, reading, eating out, taking walks, entertaining, work, and driving. Angel, for example, has withdrawn from nearly all her socializing activities, except her bridge club: "As you can imagine, that is difficult when you have got, when your hands swell. But friends are very good. They shuffle for me, they deal for me. All I've got [to do] is to hold the cards and play them. I mean I hate sort of displaying hands like this, but you know, it's another adjustment." Yet her overall account of illness suggests this is not "just another adjustment" for Angel. She has had to systematically give up the things that she has developed over the years as means for relaxation and relating to people. She has had to give up a manifestation of whom she sees herself as being.

> I used to go in there twice a month [at the charitable society], I was one of the volunteers there that ran the office. And I loved doing that. But I can't get up

there. I am too unreliable. Some days, when I get up I feel so terrible that I just go from my bed to my sofa. And I won't do anything, but I've got to do something. . . . [I]t bothers me because essentially—I remember telling my family doctor once that it was quite normal for me to watch the television, read a book, and listen, all at the same time. And he said, "No wonder you are in such a terrible state." And I hadn't thought of it like that, you know. But I was one of those people. I was, I did all sorts of things. I made my own necklaces and all that sort of thing, you know. I mean I was always, and of course up until the time I came out here, I was heavily involved in painting. I tried to paint when I came out, but I couldn't do it anymore. And that was partly because of my hands.

Angel's losses are frustrating for her. She describes herself as a "wreck." Although 76, where many women would attribute declining activities to aging, Angel directly relates her having to give up activities to RA. Even though onset of RA was more than forty years ago, Angel is still being pulled into the commonsense notion that she was trying to take on too much for too long. Being a "wreck," for Angel at least, has been justified by a (male) physician who extracts her bodily symptoms and reassigns "blame" for being a "wreck" back on her.

For women with chronic illness, having been used to a particular set of bodily activities and then being forced to give them up because of illness is problematic for sense of self.[4] Shelagh sums up her experiences as "I've lost me."

And I think what hurts me the most about this is that I've lost me. I've lost a sense of who I am and I don't know who I'm going to be anymore. And that is horrible. I mean all your life you grow up who you are and you make your plans, and some come out and some don't but you are going on the way. . . . I can't remember being that person and I don't know if it's unrealistic to think I'll ever be that person again. I know I'm not going to die of this, I know this will pass, but I don't know who I'm going to be at the end of it. And whether it would be good for me or not to go back into that extremely stressful situation [of work], I don't know yet. A small part of my heart is accepting. No, I think that day when you are better, when that comes, maybe you're going to do something else. . . . I've lost me. I've lost my life, my social life, my relationship with my husband. So no wonder I'm mad sometimes and no wonder I cry sometimes.

Shelagh expresses well the constitutive process of identity where she is rooted in her "previous" self and moving toward some as yet unknown, shapeless "new" self. The certainty of her life has disappeared to be replaced with an unstable present and ambiguous future.

This sense of a lost future resonates with the experiences of other women with chronic illness. The uncertainty associated with chronic illness confounds the women's desire to face the uncertainty of the future. The losses that women with chronic illness identify and grieve are integral to the constitutive processes of self, through which "new" identities emerge, ones focused on the self rather than on other people. As Caron points out, "Now I've reinvented myself and so I think being more aware of my own needs rather than trying to always meet others'. And so I suppose, you could say, I have become more selfish." Expressing how one was different prior to onset and recognizing how an ill body is part of an identity was important for the women. As Reann maintains, this journey to a "new" self is arduous and proceeds unevenly.

> I've only had one person from my old life, when I was well, that remained in my new life. So, that was pretty hard at the time, when there was all these friends, I was losing all these friends. But since I've just kind of stuck with it instead of getting too withdrawn, which a lot of people do, that I just made new friends. And so I have better friends now. True friends, I think. It was a couple of years of transition and some—it was pretty painful. With all these people who you thought would understand when you started falling apart, you were just too slow for them. You couldn't go for walks, you couldn't do this, you couldn't do that. And so they just stopped calling. In a way that takes the pressure off and that reduces a lot of the anxiety, is not trying to live in a, in speed that everybody else was living.

These "new" identities are not always the clean breaks that Brie talked about or the reinventions Caron mentioned. The comparative discussion of self in the periods just prior and after onset around transition, loss, and the potential for renewal indicate the ways women negotiated their ill identity discursively and materially through their own embodiment. Just as onset of illness propelled women into a destabilization of their material bodies, onset also impelled women to become cognizant of their identities *as women*. Their "previous" identities were no longer applicable because now they were *women with chronic illness*. And, although we were interested in the experiences of chronic illness, nearly all of the women refused the discursive category of ill or disabled as their only or even primary expression of identity. Stories of their experiences show how illness—with bodily limits—became constitutive of self. Like a genealogy of an individual identity, each woman could readily identify bits and pieces of her own self in the woman she had become with the experience of chronic illness. Yet the illness is there, even if not showcased, for, as Fern so aptly put it, "I have moved away. It's seven years from waking up in the morning and thinking I've got this disease and how am I going to manage today, to knowing that it is within my body, but it is not the foremost thought."

NEGOTIATING IDENTITY

In focusing in on the process through which "new" identities emerge for women with chronic illness, we have slighted attention to the friction arising from competing and contradictory inscriptions of illness and other discourses that shape women's identities. We turn now to looking at specific instances where multiple aspects of women's identities are held in tension, creating space for women to mediate power imbued in multiple sets of social relations.

Inge negotiates the tension between being ill and meeting the expectations society has of being a woman. She makes the point that being rooted in gendered expectations of women's activity gets more complicated at onset of chronic illness. "Getting hooked up on the way I was trained to operate as a woman, I could no longer operate that way once I developed arthritis. But that was all right, because a woman does not need to operate that way. So, you know, I guess in terms of my [self] image, my image was okay before, but it's better now." Inge's negotiation of the intersection of being a woman and of being ill apparently permitted her to deal with the deep-seated notions of the expectations of womanhood. Even though she appears to be comfortable with her newly negotiated identity, she went on to talk of the changes in her relationship with her husband and

> I think my husband was happier when he had a wife who took care of him more. Happier, and I mean, he is thrilled now that I am, that I managed, in that I don't have a lot of pain, and there are certain things that I can do. He's thrilled. He really is. But he—his mother took care of everything. He was married before, he was married to a woman who took care of everything, including polishing shoes. And it was very difficult to be married to him. Not that I had compassion for him—anybody who can't polish their shoes is in trouble. But it's been tough for him. He's had to learn, and it's not been easy. And he also has a fantasy of the way life is, and—which is different from the way life really is.

This hearkening back to expectations of and for women through her relationship with her husband is more of a way to "solidify," at least momentarily, or perhaps even to "justify," her newly articulated self. She is "managing" her illness and is feeling better about who she has come to be.

Just as Fern destabilized her own identity as primarily one of *being* chronically ill by "moving away" from scrutinizing her body daily, Ronnie subverted the notion that "a person with disabilities" is necessarily central to a chronically ill woman's identity. She has had RA since she was a child and uses a motorized wheelchair as her primary mobility aid. Ronnie used to be employed as a contract manager, a job that has little continuity for once a contract ends, there is no further professional contact. This type of job creates an isolation for which many women are not prepared. In Ronnie's case, this proved extremely difficult after the break up with her partner.

> I haven't worked long enough in any one place to really develop long friend-ships. When I was with my partner, I didn't feel I needed that, which is sad 'cause that was totally devastating. I was actually in a lesbian relationship. I've tried making friends in the lesbian community, going out with them. I find that extremely hard. They seem to sexualize everything and it's just, it hasn't been possible to make friendships. One gal still calls and I haven't seen her since last summer, you know, she can't work it into her schedule to meet for lunch. So, you know? And then just one other person I keep in touch with as a friend.

Ronnie negotiates several tensions—being disabled, being chronically ill, being a woman, being lesbian—all of which position her socially and politi-cally as a "body in context." It is her particular mediation of power expressed through these tensions that creates her *specific* body, one quite lonely and not comfortable within either the disability or lesbian community.[5]

Margie, too, feels disconnected from the community for persons with dis-abilities. Through encouragement from her family and friends, Margie took an office job with a resource center for persons with disabilities. She said she hated it there because she was not able to use the skills she had trained for. She felt more comfortable in a workplace where people valued her skills whether or not her employer was disabled. Although Margie did not frame her discussion of that particular job in terms of assumptions people make about persons in wheelchairs, later in her story, she discussed assumptions people make about wheelchair users around expressions of sexuality. She noted that most people "just think of a disabled person as non-sexual."

Carolyn elaborated on this theme in her general discussion about the assumptions people make about the identity of a woman using a wheelchair.

> When you are in a wheelchair there is a whole set of assumptions, I think, about people thinking that you are less competent, and usually if I'm with somebody, a lot of times people will talk to the other person that I'm with. So it gets really bad because I always speak whether they are looking at me or not. But then when they are actually talking to the other person, I often answer too, and that's really not good. It gets to be a habit. So anyway, that's one thing. I think being a woman is also an assumption, but I think mostly it's the disability thing. That has a bigger impact I think than whether I'm female or not because to tell you the truth I think a lot of people think you are asexual when you are disabled. They just don't see your gender much.

Carolyn makes an important point about repetition: "it gets to be a habit" responding to people who do not look at you when speaking. This repetition affects the expression of identity as well as notion of self. Carolyn attributes her experience of being continually dismissed in conversation because she uses a wheelchair not because she is female. Her explanation is based not on discrimination against persons with disabilities, but on the invisibility of gender and sexuality for persons with disabilities. This explanation speaks to Margie's experiences, but in a different way.

> I was really taken aback, because no other guy has ever really talked to me about, you know, relationships or anything. I think they look at me like a—you know, it's like I'm a sister kind of thing. But he said once, "Do you have a boyfriend?" And I said no, and he said, why not or whatever—you know, just the usual small talk, and then I said, oh, I just, the disabled guys that I've met, it's, I haven't liked, or it just hasn't worked out. And he said, oh, "Do you limit it to just disabled guys?" And I just about, I was floored. It showed me that he's obviously, has no—you know, realizes that we are not asexual or whatever.

Margie, through repetitive social practices, had understood that most people outside her own circle of female friends or outside of those who have extensive experience with persons with disabilities assumed disabled people were asexual. That this man asked about relationships shook Margie's understanding of her own identity, as well as the collective identity of persons with disabilities, because she, too, was part of the reproduction of disability as genderless and asexual.

Negotiating identity also involves sorting through *how* it is a woman with chronic illness wants to be chronically ill. Resolution for many of the women came through their involvement with a support group at some point in time. Leeza even started one when she lived in an area where there were very few resources. Nearly all the support groups for RA in Vancouver and Victoria are associated with institutionalized clinics devoted solely to arthritis. Nearly all of the support groups for ME are completely volunteer, self-help, and not part of institutionalized health services. For women with RA, the support groups were steadily supportive whereas for women with ME, support groups became less useful once some time had passed. With RA, the progression of the disease is problematic and women tend to need ongoing support. As well, referral to centers devoted to arthritis and their support groups is routine after diagnosis of any arthritis. With ME, the most intense part of the illness is near the beginning when women have little access to knowledge and resources about the illness. Once women begin to understand ME, or get used to coping with the unpredictability of their bodies, they stop going to support groups.[6]

We think that being part of support groups assists in the move from being healthy toward being ill—neither place being static or complete. This movement also involves shifting from being an individual with chronic illness to being a group of women who are chronically ill. Being part of any support group is a statement about being part of a larger, collective identity, a further dimension of being a "body in context." From the accounts of support group participation of the women in this study, it seems to us that women with RA identify with being ill on a longer-term basis than women with ME, who identify with being ill at some times but not at others. Support groups are but one means through which to express an identity as a woman with chronic illness. Janice, for example, illustrates this in her discussion of why she has no interest in joining a support group for women with ME.

> Zero interest because, no, because I know that I am doing better than many people. Like I know, I have one friend who is severely disabled. You know, she has not worked for eight years, she's had to move back in with her parents, I mean we are talking getting out of bed and taking a shower wrecking her for a day. And I don't want to sit with people like that. Well, for one thing, again, I mentioned that the community I am part of is so supportive.

> Interviewer: That's your church group?

> Janice: Yes. And my school. Those are very supportive groups. And I am so much of an organizer and stuff that if I went to that group, I think I might feel that I have to be politically active. And I just don't want it. And I've also, I mean I read a little bit of the literature. I try to read books about chronic fatigue. Like this *Osler's Web*,[7] and articles. I am very interested in that. But the few ME bulletins and stuff that I've read, they are so whiney I find, and so angry, and maybe it's justified when some people's entire lives have been ruined. . . . I'm just kind of bored with it, to tell you the truth. When I have conversations with them, that's all they want to talk about. So, what symptoms do you have? And it's a big enough factor in my life that I just need to be a whole person and, like it feels different to talk to you than it does to talk to them.

Janice clearly does not want to be labeled as "disabled," nor does she want her illness to be forefront in how she expresses who she is. She is supported in her economic privilege and even though she feels poorly and is unable to teach full-time, she refuses to be part of a collective identity of being ill.

DISCLOSURE

Integral to the constitution of identity is the issue of disclosure. Publicly claiming a diagnosis of chronic illness means publicly claiming being ill, something which is difficult to do for a number of reasons, the fear of losing an able identity, a comfortably articulated self, and "me" being most common, with many women also expressing fear of losing work and being discriminated against in the workplace. Ruth decided not to disclose her diagnosis of RA to anyone in the workplace initially because "I was expecting it all to go away. Give it a couple of months and I will feel better." Ruth had just begun a small cleaning business with a friend, "and I thought, this suits me, we'll see if we can make this work. I don't have to leave town. And it was working. It had been about four or five months that I'd been working." Eventually Ruth was forced to disclose because of the increasing constraints on her bodily movements from the progression of the disease. Many of the women had similar experiences—keeping the diagnosis and illness to themselves rather than disclosing to employers, friends, and coworkers.

Disclosure is not only about revealing illness in the workplace, it is also about revealing chronic illness socially, thus legitimating the set of activities comprising what it is to be ill. For many women with chronic illness, symptoms are invisible. Another person cannot "see" pain, fatigue, or cognitive impairment. It is only through interaction that illness comes to be known by others, and sometimes only through astute observation during interaction, because women try to hide the fact that they are not "normal." For women with chronic illness, this invisibility is closely linked to denial of experience because of the importance western culture places on visual legitimacy. The validity of being ill is challenged when disclosure of illness produces no visible support for such a claim.

Being denied as ill has implications for a sense of self, and as Alex puts it, it makes one feel "like a fraud, like a sham. Like a lazy person." It also affects how to express illness publicly. Alex describes her experiences of being denied in terms of not appearing to be ill. She has been called a "lady of leisure" and "lucky" not to have to work. These types of comments make her angry because people are not taking the time to understand ME and how the illness affects her life.

> And they don't understand that if I wash the car, that's it. That is my whole day. There is no more. The chances are I won't cook dinner and I will do nothing else for the rest of the day. It just, oh you know, I see you out doing such and such, you must be feeling better. But you did nothing the day before because you knew you had to go out that day, you had to rest up. . . . I guess it's a little bit hurtful because you want to be the way you used to be and you want to be normal, active, healthy, happy whatever.

This tension between wanting to be "normal" and wanting to be accepted *as is* (at a given time) plays itself out differently in the context of disclosure for individual women with chronic illness. It leads to frustration for many women, and limited social interaction. Personal relationships may dissolve. Public disclosure sometimes leads to situations in which women with chronic illness are forced to abandon their previous notions of self in relation to "bodies in context," and negotiate "new" identities more in keeping with their reconstituted self.

For women with ME, their reactions to negative experiences of public disclosure were more intense, more piercing, and more dismissive than for women with RA. Invalidation for women with ME is a common occurrence. Because women with ME often are not visibly ill[8] or do not have a completely sound biomedical diagnosis, they frequently are not treated as if they are ill, which has repercussions for the way they see themselves. Connie contrasted the way people had responded to her experience of breast cancer and later her experiences with ME. When she underwent surgery to remove both breasts, her coworkers were sympathetic, lavished her with attention, and wished her well. A few years later, when she went on sick leave with ME, she did not receive the same attention or well-wishing. Breast cancer is acute, popularly known, and biomedically high profile, and it is known that if not properly treated, it can cause death. With ME being so nebulous, women diagnosed with ME continually question themselves about being ill. Brie makes these distinctions in her discussion of disclosure. "But for many it's very puzzling, and for oneself as well, and so yes, you don't—there's not much you can see. I think if you could say, well, you know—horrid thing to say, but you know, I think if you have cancer, everybody, you know, my God. You know. It's a terrible thing."

For women with ME, distinguishing the difference between "being tired" and being ill with ME is important because the distinction is central to their identity as a woman with chronic illness. Brie, continuing her discussion of public perceptions of different types of illness, indicates that being ill with ME is a *specific* identity, one that can be easily identifiable if *specific* meanings are expressed, those arising out of *specific* experiences of the body.

But if you say something—I mean, even the name's so unfortunate. Fatigue. Like I sometimes, I remember, I told a couple of people, and the response is, well, you know, you're getting older. We all have off days. And, you know, we all feel a bit down at times. You know, I can't do as much as I used to. And you think, oh, forget it. Tired is a normal response. This other fatigue is not that, whatever it used to, to me it feels electrical. It's sort of like when the battery's gone dead. Or it's overworked, you're all electrified and on edge, sparking all over the place and you can't stop it. But mostly you're just—the battery's dead. So, you know, that was the sort of frame of reference. That it's the cells and the nerves seem, you know, burnt out, and—it's nothing to do with feeling tired. So of course when you talk to people in the frame of reference of it's tiredness. . . . *You know, unless you've been through it, you're in another frame of reference.*

We mark Brie's last words because framing experiences in ways that can be understood by others is what diagnosing illness is about. And when most people are existing in another frame of reference, such as physicians, insurance adjusters, family members, friends, grocery store clerks, strangers, or neighbors, then women with ME become invalid whether or not they disclose their illness. If they claim to have ME, they are challenged; when they don't, their bodily limits reveal themselves as incompetent, unable, and limited. Brie goes on to elaborate on what she means as "frame of reference" as a way to place into context the circumstance within which something constitutes an act as an experience.

> Other people don't talk the language, 'cause even the doctors are debating. How do we take this? I used to say to my friend, put me in a room and let me talk to people and I can tell you if they have it or not. You have a common language. You know, you can tell by—you know, that they're brain dead. You know, I left my brain on the pillow today. It's gone again. . . . As I say, if I meet someone, I can usually tell in a few minutes—sometimes it's a borderline and I don't know. But often I can say, no way. They can be allergies, whatever. But they have the basic language.

MOVING TOWARD EVERYDAY LIFE

It is probably unfair to use the analogy of transition to describe the constitutive processes of self and identity for women with chronic illness. Within the concept of transition there is the implied notion that there exists another state of being at the end of the transition, as a closure to one's struggles and tribulations. This really is not the case for women with chronic illness. As the accounts of women's experiences of chronic illness here show, waxing and waning of bodily limits and borders of illness create spaces where women form a sense of self and negotiate their identities. The fleeting specific articulations of temporary identities and the unpredictability of bodily being become ways of life. Long term, when dealing with chronicity, does not equal stability in expressions of self, identity, and predictability of illness; rather, long term brings with it a delicate complacency with being in an ongoing unstable, unpredictable transition. Underlying the expression of *specific* identities after onset of illness is the absence of presence and the presence of absence. Paramount in the negotiation of an ill identity for these women with chronic illness was the notion that there was no "present" in their lives. Most of the women discussed their "previous" life and how they would like to see themselves in the future, with very few women framing their stories as being themselves as they are now. Many women dealt with this absence of a presence by asserting their desire to be present *as is*, however that may be. In order to affirm who it is they were at any point in time in a particular place, they found it necessary to deal with the presences of absences. Through grieving their losses, they were able to sort through some aspects of their illness in relation to self. Embodying the fluid borders of illness gives women with chronic illness room to negotiate identity through mediating the power imbued in the social relations they engage in and reassert themselves as women with chronic illness into the prevailing deployment of power/knowledge/space. Expressing these transitory identities, incomplete ones that fluctuate in time and across space, means structuring and restructuring corporeal spaces of everyday life. Transition for women with chronic illness has no preferred end state of being; transition is about being *as is,* somewhere between what they used to be and how they will be in the future.

9

Disciplining the Environment through Re-learning the Body: Everyday Life, Minutiae, Daily Living

She's going to be mad. I shouldn't have taken that nap. If I hurry. I can't hurry that much. Got my keys. Got my purse. Do I need anything else? Money. Yes, I've got money. . . . The phone. Maybe it's Danielle. Do I answer it? I'd better. Ross. Not now, I don't have time. Please, please, don't talk anymore. This week-end. Right. "I can't go this weekend. It just isn't going to work out." *Okay. Okay. Yes. I know.* "I've got to go. I'm picking up Danielle. I'll tell her you phoned." *. . . Now I'm really going to be late. . . . Why does he do that? Phone in the middle of the day to tell me stuff that he knows will just make me angry. I don't need to know his schedule. . . . Wait a minute, maybe he was telling me that I wouldn't have to go because he was going to Ladysmith with Danielle. I need to pay more attention. It seems as if I lost everything. My Dad. My friends. My husband. And now he's getting married. . . . Routine. Routine. That's what I need. If only I could remember everything. Then I'd know what to expect. . . . This traffic. What time is it? Oh no! . . .* "Sorry I'm late, honey. I got caught up on the phone." *Please don't get upset.* "With your Dad." *. . . That wasn't too bad. Maybe she won't mind that I won't be going.* "So, how was your day?" *. . . Wow. She's busy. I wonder how this "thing" with my body is affecting her? It's never clear. But it's got to bother her. And, Ross, too. He's so annoying. . . . I need to take another nap. What am I thinking? Routine. Right. I can't have routine. I have this body! . . . I've got to get an answering machine.*

Situating identity, subjectivity, and experience in spatial contexts assist in elaborating the notion of spatiality. If the spatial and the social are forever

145

entwined, each within the other, then identity inevitably has to be spatial and the spatial is inescapably a part of subjectivity. Pulling out the spatial aspects of women living with chronic illness, as we have argued before, may sound hackneyed and a little clichéd. Changes to such a routine to accommodate bodily limits, such as aligning the bed with a clear path to the bathroom or perhaps cutting out socializing in the evenings, sound like common sense. But because of the repetitiveness of everyday life comprised of elements of the mundane that make our lives routine, women with chronic illness sometimes overlook "the obvious," and struggle with their physical surroundings and social relationships.

Making sense of living with chronic illness means embracing *notions* and *practices* associated with volatility. Not only are the bodies of women with chronic illness volatile, so are the spaces they traverse. For example, depending on the context of the people in a workplace, the woman's employment *vis-à-vis* her coworkers and employer, and the policies in place for women with chronic illness, the workplace could either be supportive or exclusive. Those supportive take on volatility and provide flexible working conditions in terms of tasks, workload, and equipment; those exclusive reject the precariousness of the woman and her work and demand that she perform as she always had, prior to onset of illness. Accepting volatility entails redefining flare-ups and remissions, "good" days and "bad" days, as daily occurrences, disrupting the trajectory of a woman's search to "be cured" or to "return to normal." Redefining volatility as daily occurrence reframes the minutiae of everyday life and claims corporeal spaces as unstable, unpredictable, and uncertain. Through this embodied volatility, women with chronic illness continue to negotiate tensions between reliance and independence, between order and chaos, between health and illness.

Through the process of adjusting to the unpredictability of everyday life with their own volatile bodies, women relinquish control over their bodies. By relinquishing control, we do not mean that women cease to treat the physiological and biological aspects of the chronic illness or that women deny the materiality of their body. Rather, we suggest that women with chronic illness adjust to the undulating pulses of bodily pain, fatigue, and cognitive impairment so as to make sense of their illness, moving through time and space with these rhythmic vibrations instead of continually fighting against them. Moving with bodily pulsations, through time and space, provides women with the opportunity to intervene in the constitutive processes of identity and effect some sort of change. The experiences of the women we discussed in the previous chapters indicate some possibilities of how women with chronic illness shape their own "ill" identities, through encounters with medical professionals, family members and friends, and employers and coworkers. For women with chronic illness, intervention into these constitutive processes can also play out through asserting control over everyday spaces—living, working, and clinical environments. By asserting control, we mean a range of activities that restructure physical and social aspects of these environments in their quest to make sense of their (discursive and material) bodily limits while existing in the borders of illness and health. Engaging these activities in effect *disciplines* the environment and redefines what it is to be ill.

This disciplining of the environment permeates all aspects of everyday life—from the most mundane act to the most extraordinary event—affecting the spatial organization of surrounding environments and the timing of each seemingly insignificant undertaking. The circumscription of environments by time and space sets the parameters for how to go about intervening into the processes constitutive of spatialities. Women with chronic illness engage these parameters and structure their immediate spaces and the timing of activities so that they are able to complete a certain set of daily living and working tasks on their terms. This engagement "on their own terms" is the crux of disciplining the environment—women with chronic illness must re-learn their bodies, discursively and materially, and pull together what it means to engage their immediate environments on their own terms. Through this process of *re-cognition*, women with chronic illness become acutely aware of their own embodiment within corporeal space—the living spaces of "bodies in context." Disciplining the environment is not a coping strategy; it is a re-working of *being*. For women with chronic illness, this means being ill and healthy, discursively and materially, at the same time.

One way to understand women's experiences of the fluid borders of chronic illness is to scrutinize the stories of women's descriptions of their everyday lives. Through these depictions of their environments, women with chronic illness express temporal and spatial specificities of their own volatile bodies. In claiming to be *as is* within their own corporeal spaces, women with chronic illness patently embrace their volatility and gain access to the social and spatial processes constituting their identity and subjectivity. Disciplining the environment is predicated upon the notion of volatility, and, once volatility is accepted in everyday life, new understandings of experience emerge, ones that can transform bodily activities in ways that undermine hegemony and challenge prevailing deployments of power/knowledge/space. In the rest of this chapter, we show how women with chronic illness *discipline* the environment as part of the constitutive processes of spatiality. We first draw out examples of the extensive changes in social networks women with chronic illness face after onset of illness. Next we demonstrate how the re-cognition of the body forces women to acknowledge how the immediacy of their own corporeal space is imbued with matter, meanings, and emotions. In our discussion of what might comprise usual, daily activities in the life of a woman with chronic illness, we query the notion of a typical day, emphasizing the volatility and uncertainty of bodies and spaces. Finally, we show in more detail how the body transforms from a steady entity through which women learn to make sense of their surrounding environments into an unsure one, through which women must re-learn both themselves and their environments.

DEPARTURE POINTS AND BELONGINGS

Women with chronic illness create, then designate, a departure point for negotiating everyday life. Many women with chronic illness use aspects of spirituality as a departure point for sorting through what they believe about illness and how their body is integrated into the notion of who they are. Even for those women where spirituality was not central in their lives (through, for example, meditation or prayer), accessing inner sanctums of contemplation was important to begin healing—not from the illness itself; rather, from the onset of illness. Rhonda recounts a conversation she had with a friend about "inner healing," who challenged her about having accepted RA as part of who she was.

> But this holistic doctor friend, also, he asked me a couple of questions. He said, "Have you accepted the fact that you have RA?" And I said, "Yes, I think I have." And he said, "Have you learned anything from it?" And I thought about it and I said, "A lesson for me has been that I can live a very happy life without having to do all the things I thought I had to be able to do. And part of that is not needing to work full time. And not needing to be the biggest, best, fastest, more, whatever."
>
> Interviewer: Superwoman.
>
> Rhonda: Exactly. . . . He said, "Have you given thanks for it?" I said, "No. I can say that I have not given thanks for it." And we talked about it in terms of a reductionist model of illness and health and a more holistic model of illness and health. I don't know if you've read some of this stuff. But the whole idea that illness is something. Your body is letting you down. It's something you have got to try and get rid of. It's all these negative things. Versus illness as something which is an opportunity for learning. Your body might be dying to tell you something. So that's another reason for me wanting to go looking at some of this inner, personal growth, healing stuff. Because I think there is obviously something to be learned there. And I would still, overall, because in another question he asked, he said, "Can you picture yourself being healthy and still having rheumatoid arthritis?" And at first I said yes, provided I stay in remission. Haven't got any symptoms. That's not exactly being accepting of what's going on in the moment. So I'm just thinking about some of those ideas.

Rhonda frames her challenge as one of being able to look at RA, not as a disease that needs only to be controlled, but she wants to be able to take on having RA as a state of being, or as she says, being healthy and still having RA—even when it is not in remission.

Women with chronic illness often cannot take on this "inner work" without already having in place a supportive social network. Identity, illness, and context together constitute corporeal space—supportive relationships are part of that milieu. So even if a woman has a supportive network of family members and friends at onset, this does not guarantee that such support continues. Many of the women we talked with lost friends primarily because of expectations of activity levels. For example, if the women had related to a friend through sport, like tennis, hiking, windsurfing, or jogging, then the friendship was in peril. As Pauline noted, the "depth" of friendships change. "I used to have more interesting friends, or I used to—friends that were doing more. That doesn't necessarily make them more interesting, but—I used to have friends that were more active and more involved in the world, and, you know, doing this and that. Playing more roles in the world. Now my friends tend to be more retiring introverted types, more like I am now." This shift influences the women's approach to understanding their own daily life and shapes their responses. Caron explains this process in more detail.

> I only have one friend that the friendship almost died I think because she has real difficulty when people are ill. It's almost like she is personally offended that you are not there to do the things with her. And she would, at the beginning, she would say things like if you would just take up jogging, why don't you take up running, why don't you go out and play tennis. I sort of explained I cannot do that and then she got really annoyed and it was almost as though she thought I was making it all up. After about a year she actually said to me, "You know, I think I've been in denial. I just didn't like the way that you were sick and I realized that you really are sick."

Pauline and Caron, like many of the other women, tend to measure friendships after onset in terms of understanding and support. This act of measuring assists the women in creating a supportive space so that she can begin to heal.

Living in the borders of illness has an impact on negotiating spaces of everyday life. Women with chronic illness face the tension between wanting to belong and be included in activities beyond those they may be capable of intermittently and desiring to be alone to engage in activities that will promote a sense of wellness. Debby expresses this negotiation in terms of not wanting to "miss out on something," but not wanting to feel worse physically. "So, you know, I would really like to, and especially when [my friends] all get together with each other out there or whatever, on long weekends or whatever. Then I feel like, oh yeah, I'm really missing out on something. But I get kind of sick of saying no, but I don't feel bad at all. No, that's tough luck for them, I mean, I'm doing the best I can." She goes on to point out that most of her friends, although recognizing that ME is actually an illness and not "in her head," do not work through the ramifications of what having ME means in terms of daily living.

> But it's like, oh, why can't you come over, well, with three little kids running around I'd just come home exhausted, that's why I'm not coming over. But you know, they just don't quite get that, because they're just not in my position. . . . You know, they come here and I look fine, I probably look fine to you too, and they leave and I'm sure they kind of scratch their heads going "Hum, what's going on with that girl?" But again it's just something I just put out at arm's length. If they can't figure it out, I, you know, I—that's their problem. I can't spend my whole time trying to convince them. Why, I mean, I just, kind of selfish in that way, because I'm looking after myself first.

In her story, Debby pinpoints the intersection of illness, identity, and corporeal space as the departure point for negotiating her everyday life. The living spaces of being ill matter in ways that can transform how a woman with chronic illness is ill. Engaging in education around ME is important, but not central to either the desire to belong or to receive support. Debby sets limits that are flexible, depending on the friend or the place, to her corporeal space within which she can maneuver while ill.

DISCIPLINING THE ENVIRONMENT IN LIEU OF BODILY CONTROL

Setting limits to corporeal space initiates the process of disciplining the environment. These limits expand and contract according to the displays of the embodiment of women with chronic illness. Constitutive of corporeal space are material bodies and physical surroundings, meanings associated with bodies and places, and emotions. Whereas materiality and meaning grant substance to spatiality, it is the expression of emotions that provide the garish texture. Nicola discussed how stress affects how she is able to be ill in particular places.

> Well, I think the home environment, I've realized through my life that the home environment, work environment, whatever environment, that the more tension and the more aggravation that there is there, the sicker I am. Even when I was, didn't have the arthritis, that was true for me. My body can't, because of my background, and I was not allowed to feel anything, so I would put all of my emotions into my body. And today, that is still true to some

extent. And with the arthritis, it's only intensified that. I can't sit in a room where two people are arguing and not get stiff. It's taken me a long time to realize the connection. . . . But I realize still that I can't handle some conflicts, especially a man and woman fighting.

Nicola's knowledge of how the intensity of emotion can affect the body shapes her response to RA. Having already been sensitized to the corporeality of tension arising from conflict, she understands the significance of the (constitutive) interaction of emotion and space. Recognizing stress and responding by changing immediate living spaces, sometimes by simply leaving a room, is one way to intervene in the process of structuring space and de-link self from what a woman perceives as being an unhealthy environment.

This description of a minute negotiation of corporeal space reveals how a woman with chronic illness might go about disciplining the environment at any scale. These negotiations, however, could be long, drawn-out sets of activities, often complicated by intense feelings of isolation. Furthermore, because of the unpredictability of illness itself, women were often unable to plan ahead for small or large social events. And, if they did make plans, as Debby spoke about, the women sometimes unwillingly broke commitments. The material limits of the body set parameters for social interaction, limited mobility during flare-ups, environmental sensitivities and allergies in public places, and ongoing fatigue. Limited income also *severely* restricts what types of activities women with chronic illness can engage in, ranging from taking vacations to meeting for coffee, from phoning long distance to going to the movies. Women with chronic illness tend not to travel on vacation, will drink coffee at home, wait for friends from afar to phone, and often watch videos.

In order to deal with the tension between wanting to be alone and feeling isolated and left out, women with chronic illness engage in quite specific practices. Most practices included some form of closing off social contacts, minimizing interaction, and continuous monitoring of bodily aptness. Yvonne successfully used the telephone as a way to forge friendships and seek therapy. Jayne bartered with her daughter and neighbors over gardening and housework. Charlotte, Stella, and Renee kept a "things to do" list by the kitchen door, awaiting family members to come by and help. Formal support networks are beneficial for some women. Support groups can also be lifelines to women isolated by their illness. Teresa is involved with four different groups for people with vertigo, agoraphobia, Fibromyalgia, and ME. She formed several supportive friendships via telephone contacts through these groups. This is important for Teresa because she lost several friends at the onset of her illness and is estranged from her family. Renee slowly built her network up from nothing. Prior to her illness, her primary social network was an athletic group, where she was a trainer. She moved with her husband to the Maritimes where the onset of RA occurred. She was unemployed without any social support, recovering from a fall associated with RA, and her husband left her without any money. It took her two years to get enough money to move back to Victoria. But she could not connect to her old network there, and had to forge new friendships and relationships. It was quite difficult given her bodily limitations. Her friends now consist solely of women with chronic illness—quite a variety of illnesses. It is easy to see the body as a site of resistance when seeing these women build social networks in spite of being ill. These women restructure their environments to accommodate their disabling illness, to create a corporeal space through which they feel they belong and have some connection with others.

Outside the minutiae of everyday life, during "extraordinary" events of daily living, women with chronic illness and those that are supportive of them strive to resist the intrusions of non-supportive matter, meanings, and emotions in order to control their corporeal spaces. Barbara and Janice were two of the few women who gave birth while ill. Barbara said that she felt physically better with regard to the RA while pregnant, even though after each pregnancy the RA worsened. Eventually Barbara hired a live-in nanny to assist her in caring for her three young children. Janice's experience of pregnancy, childbirth, and childrearing were nearly the opposite of Barbara—her symptoms intensified while pregnant and, after the birth of her second child, she struggled to raise her children on her own while her husband worked. Janice's most vivid description of her corporeal space around the time of pregnancy was the period of time just before delivery. She was terribly anxious to give birth. This anxiety was compounded by lack of sleep. She was finally reassured once her physician revealed her plan to induce labor.

> So that, at least there would be a day that I could know that this would be the day that he would be born. But of course I found this out on Thursday and I was supposed to come in on Monday. I didn't have any idea how to get through Friday, Saturday, and Sunday. I thought you may as well kill me. I mean, it was just so big to me. I was so tired. So, what ended up happening, what was interesting was the nurse that was with me on the day when I had this IV, I was still able at that point to remain fairly, like I could keep the my dignity again. That's the word I use because I was aware. I separated myself in my mind. Like there was a part of me that could remain sane and objective. And so I was this blubbering, desperate woman.

Her separation of self—between a "sane and objective" woman and a "blubbering, desperate" woman—was a strategy she used to "fit" into the clinical environment of hospital while at the same time demonstrating that she needed assistance in "getting through" the last moment before birth. This separation was a way to discipline the environment *through* her self. But she was not truly comfortable with who she was at that moment. "I wouldn't even lie down on the bed because I was afraid with, I mean I was just completely gone, right? There was doctors coming and going and this nurse who had seen me two weeks earlier, I heard her say, 'I have never seen anything like this!' And those words still bother me because it wasn't me. I felt like this isn't me, but I couldn't help myself." After the birth, Janice's physician suggested that she seek out counseling for her anxiety.

> They said you should, and I had no resistance to it. . . . You know, I have no problem baring my soul to someone. So I went to a few sessions. But really, I think we had set up four and I went three and the third one was cut short. There was really nothing more to say. I mean he was excellent. He helped me to see that given all the circumstances, there was nothing odd about what had happened. You know? The panic attacks are medically explainable, but nobody told me that at the time. In fact, I didn't know what was happening. They are so frightening.

The response by her physician indicated that Janice was "out of control" during the last days of pregnancy and needed to somehow gain control over her self again. After having had her behavior "medically explained" by panic attack—another discursive category of diagnosis—Janice was able to make sense once again of her volatile body. She slid into her corporeal space, a place where she could be ill and negotiate her identity and the fluctuations of her illness as a way to discipline the environment in lieu of bodily control.

A TYPICAL DAY?

There is no doubt that the discursive and material bodily limits at the borders of illness contribute to the "shrinking" world that women with chronic illness live in. Pauline mentioned that this "shrinking" is both literal and metaphorical. Many spaces are closed off as a result of illness—schools, malls, workplaces, friends' homes, and even parts of a woman's own home—because women with chronic illness can no longer be part of them on a daily basis. Quitting school or work because the tasks are too onerous, not getting to socialize because a friend's house is too crowded or noisy, or being too fatigued to venture outside the bedroom literally preclude women with chronic illness from being in particular spaces. Such actions metaphorically rule out a "normal" life, something women with chronic illness deal with when negotiating an "ill" identity. For Debby, the link between bodily limits and a "shrinking" world is clear even within the midst of being in flux.

> Well, your world becomes very small, because it [the illness], as you learn to live with it, you find out where your limits are. And if you stay within them, you're fine. And if your limits are pretty small then you have to stay in a very—

you know what you can do and you can't do. But if you, if you set goals that you know are outside your limits, it just doesn't work.

Teresa's experiences highlight the intensity of a spatial collapse of her everyday life. After quitting her job, her husband supported her financially for several years. Throughout this period, Teresa had been imperceptibly withdrawing from social life outside her husband's sphere in order to save her energy for the deteriorating relationship. Once he left, she realized that her "world" had shrunk considerably. Like Renee, she was left in a position where she had to structure a supportive environment from scratch. At onset of RA, Eve, as part of facilitating the congealing of a blended family, lived in a house with nine offset levels. After a year of continuing to do all the housework, including the gardening, budgeting, and parenting, while ill, she and her family moved to a one-level rancher, a place more accommodating to her limited mobility. By shifting places of residence, Eve was able to reconstitute her immediate living space so that she had space and time to be ill. Both of these examples depict spatial collapses of shrinking worlds due to illness, and, like many women with chronic illness, they turned to disciplining the environment as a strategy to affect the constitution of illness and identity. Both examples indicate the *flexibility* of restructuring the physical and social aspects of the environments of daily living.

Eluding the instability of the borders of illness, the uncertainty of volatile bodies, and the constitutive spaces of identity in their daily living is not possible for women with chronic illness. Descriptions of the everyday lives the women we talked with provided us were rich in detail, but inevitably incomplete. Requesting an account of a "typical day" is a common way to get at the minutiae that makes up daily living. As we talked with, listened to the recordings, and read the transcripts of the interviews, we realized that the incompleteness of day-to-day accounts of living was not due to being sidetracked. We initially thought that the incompleteness of descriptions of a typical day was due to the inconsistency in interview styles of the four interviewers. However, after scrutinizing the transcripts, we came to understand two things: that the typicality of daily living for women with chronic illness needs to be challenged and that the accounts themselves are volatile. Dolores reiterates the former point in her response to the questions, "What is a typical day for you? Or, do you have a typical day?"

I don't have a typical day. It is so different because I am not working. Like sometimes I'll have appointments. When I feel good, if it's a feel good day. If I wake up in the morning and I've actually got energy, I'm going great. I'm going to cook. I'll cook a lot so that I can, don't have to worry about the next meeting . . . or whatever the next couple of days.

Dolores differentiated between the specifics of spending her time and the way she likes to arrange her day. She continued, explaining how she asserts control over her social environment.

> But there is no such thing as a typical day because you don't know how you feel. That's the frustrating part, is that you really don't know. I've had to cancel out sometimes with my friends. I have to cut out a lot on my friends because I had to cut out a lot of my negative friends that always were bitching and complaining and you know, asking me when am I going to go back to work and stuff. So you become very choosy with whom you want to spend your quality time. And I only want to spend time with positive people. And I know I would have nice energy around me. I will stay away from, I try not to read the newspaper, anything with violence in it. I try to stay away. I try to read stuff that is sunny, you know. Because I just don't have the energy to feel.

The goal for Dolores is to discipline the environment just enough so that she has enough energy to reproduce herself on a daily basis. By invoking this type of discipline, Dolores is able to "place" herself as a "body in context" and embody her social environment.

Some of the women did provide "specifics"—extensive, detailed accounts—of what they considered a typical day. Leeza related her experiences of her daily life.

> Well, I get up at 7:30, and if there's laundry to be done I usually get the load in the machine right away, and my husband sets the table for breakfast. And so we clean up after that, and—well, then I basically, [I do] what I do, I mean I don't do much of anything. But I'll have maybe some pictures I like to get into the photo album. Or I have to go and pick up some groceries. I have to go make some copies for something or other, some articles that I've seen, and—what else do I do? Like you say, it's not anything to speak about, it's just things that kind of come up as you live, and like pictures from a trip, right, I'll try to get them in the photo album, but I can only work on that for a little while. And then our son got married, so I was working on the photo album. So you work on that if there's not much else to do, because there again I can't concentrate for very long. So I'll work on that for half an hour or an hour and put it away again. Like, that kind of thing. Photo album, that's very hard on my eyes and my head, so I'd work on that for about a half an hour or an hour and I'd have to lie down for an hour. You know. And by that time, it's lunchtime, and after that it's—usually after lunch I go for a walk. I do go for a walk every day, about twenty minutes. And that's as fast or as slow as I can handle it for that day. You know, sometimes I can go lickety-split, and other times I just slow right down. Or I might even just go halfway and come back. It all depends on how I feel. . . . So I'll do that whenever it fits in, I mean that might fit in before lunch or after lunch, or whatever I was doing in the morning. If I come back from shopping I probably have to lie down for a while. And—what happens after that? That's kind of middle of the afternoon

then, it's time to start thinking about supper. I have a cup of tea and sit down for a little while. Maybe read for a little while, or, then suppertime, and after supper I've kind of had it. Then—I will sit and read for a while after supper, some light relaxing stuff. I mean I do enjoy reading deep things, I mean that's my pleasure to do that, but I can't do that right now. That's another thing I've had to stop, because my brain just won't absorb it. I read something really interesting and deep, and I can read that for maybe about ten or fifteen minutes, and then I just, you know, my brain gets sore and tired and I just have to stop. But then I can still pick up like a *Reader's Digest* or just a novel or whatever and read that for a while, I mean I can read for a couple of hours as long as I don't have to use my brain too much. So, and, well, I go to bed early, I'm in bed by 11:00. And yeah, doesn't sound like a very exciting day, but that's about the way it goes.

There are two points we want to draw out for discussion. First, Leeza repeats several times that she has been working on the photo album and that she can only work on the album for a half an hour or an hour. For us, the repetition in her narrative indicates an attempt to reproduce the mundaneness of her daily living while clarifying her bodily limits. Working on only one task before lunch might appear to signify a dreary existence. So, rather than put on display a boring itinerary, she pushes to legitimate the boundedness of her activities. Second, the seemingly itinerant mention of the photo album as a central activity of the day detracts from what she might be saying. Leeza might well have highlighted dusting, watching television, or hemming trousers; her point is that what she ends up spending most of her time doing is something that people who do not arrange their daily living environment around the accommodation of chronic illness would fit in to their lives. Instead, for Leeza, such mundane tasks become the focal point of any one day. Her claim that "I don't do much of anything," sustains her notion that the commonplace activities of everyday life are unimportant, and thus by extension her own activities too are unimportant.

This repetitive pattern appears in many of the women's stories. The "specifics" in the descriptions of what women considered typical played out differently depending on the context within which the women were embedded. Sometimes the repetition legitimated her bodily limits. At other times, the repetition signaled a shift from a justificatory move toward understanding illness as part of her lived experience—a re-cognition of her body as part of her corporeal space. Some women provided accounts of the minutiae of their daily lives in more linear narratives, primarily as part of an activity of recounting their time, reflecting on their engagement with specific sets of activities. From these types of stories, we drew a deeper understanding of the undulating circumscription of the everyday lives of women with chronic illness. Our efforts to figure out how volatile bodies exist and act in volatile environments further confirmed that a typical day is not useful as a concept if too narrowly cast or literally taken for understanding experiences of women with chronic illness. If we take volatility seriously, then typicality loses meaning. Yet the women's descriptions of what might be considered typical could be useful in understanding the women's notions of accommodating fluctuating bodies and uncertain environments. Yvonne gave two portraits of a "typical day"—the "bad" and the "good."

> Okay, well, maybe I should start with a typical bad day. I get up fairly early because most of my strength and clarity is in the morning. And I will get up and I will just start making breakfast. And I'll eat it. And then I'll have enough strength to do the dishes. And the dishes are all the previous day's . . . [interruption] . . . so I get all those done. And then it's time for my second breakfast. Usually it's an hour and half later, so by then the hypoglycemia kicks in, so I'm cooking again. When I have my second breakfast I am usually pretty tired and it's time to sit down. And I will listen to the radio, the CBC radio, a lot. And I will lie down. And by then it's lunchtime and it's time to get up and start cooking again. Often after lunch I have got to sleep. That's a pretty good day so far. Bad days, like the pattern stays pretty much the same, but there would be a lot of time spent crying and more time spent sleeping. And just feeling more emotional. I do try to get in some kind of mild exercise in a day. That would be a really good day. If I could get out somewhere to go for a walk, or to get outside into the yard and maybe do ten minutes of lawn mowing or ten minutes of weed pulling or something. That is a real accomplishment, a good thing. The afternoon is spent with very little activity. Mostly just sitting and listening to the radio or tapes that I have. Or possibly lying down. I often have appointments too, by telephone. Counseling or otherwise. And pretty much those are in the morning or in the early afternoon. Sometimes, depending on what day of the week it is, I might have to go for a grocery run. I would phone ahead and then go down and pick that up. And then by four o'clock it's time to start cooking supper. Oh, there is a mid-afternoon snack in there, too, somewhere. Around two. By four, it's time to cook supper and I spend a lot of time preparing that. It's usually over with by five or half past. And then I usually get into a real, it's time to just settle down and start doing nothing. I get in a real vegetative state after I eat dinner and the most I can do is sit and watch TV. I don't answer the phone. All contact stops after dinner. It's like my private time to just tune the world out and quit worrying about things and quit trying to accomplish anything. I sort of use TV like a drug that way. And, in between, you know, if I am feeling up for it and I want to do something else, like I might turn the TV off and do something else like go outside and water a plant, or that. But usually the rest of the evening is spent around the television set.

The extensiveness of Yvonne's discipline of her living environment is immense—she arranges her activities of daily living around her experiences of being embodied *through* her lived spaces. Although Yvonne's experiences of everyday are more tightly circumscribed than many of the other women's experiences, her story demonstrates the extent to which women with chronic illness can discipline the environment by embodying the borders of her illness. She lives alone and is responsible only for herself. She conducts most of her social interaction by phone and, because of her severe environmental allergies, limits the time she spends away from her immediate living environment. Yvonne has re-learned her body and through this re-learning has reconstituted her self as part of her corporeal space. She becomes a *specific* body.

RESTRUCTURING, RE-COGNITION, RE-LEARNING, RE- . . .

Three sites where women negotiate their identities as *specific* bodies are the clinic, the workplace, and the home. The clinic is an institutional site where disease is proclaimed or dismissed.[1] For an illness like RA, blood tests and x-rays determine the extent to which the disease is active and what damage has occurred. For an illness like ME, the interaction that takes place between the physician, patient, and diagnostic tests determines what label will be assigned to the destabilized material body.[2] Rather than revisiting the diagnosis process that we discussed in chapter 6, we would rather show how these competitive knowledges played out in the project itself. One woman with ME contacted us to ensure that we would only be talking to women actually diagnosed with ME by a biomedical physician. She thought it would taint our study if we were to talk with women who merely "thought" they had ME. Another woman had a parallel concern: she wanted us to talk only with women who had severe RA, not to women who merely had episodic flare-ups. These concerns demonstrated to us that women with chronic illness were uneasy with the possibility that their story would not be told "truthfully," that their experiences would be dismissed as not being authentic, that information as knowledge might arise from the *wrong* specific bodies. This attempt to impose parameters around what could "count" as experiences of chronic illness also shows how significant chronic illness was in their everyday lives.[3]

Jeannette's experiences show how the workplace is a site to negotiate her identity as a *specific* body. With the support of a coworker, Jeannette was able to define herself as disabled and secure financial support.

> I ended up just being grateful that I could spend some days at home to just sort of recover from that. . . . I had an open dialogue there in terms of my health because they kept pressuring me to come on full-time, and I ended up resisting that. And saying no, my health is a concern. They didn't know about it ahead of time because I was only hired on as a temporary person. And then,

when they told me they wanted me full-time, I sort of said, or permanently, I said, well, but I won't be working full-time. So they knew from the very beginning what the deal was. And they knew about my health. And in fact the woman in charge of the payroll was the one who said to me, you won't get another job that is as flexible as this in terms of your health. Take disability because you are going to be laid off because the company was sort of downsizing. . . . And so, I mean, that's the first time in my life that I had ever considered not working and having, being supported by a doctor. And I must admit, even now, I find that really difficult. I don't like even admitting it to people that I'm sort of getting sort of a disability thing.

Even though Jeannette already had a good sense of her bodily limits— spending half the week recovering from working the other half of the week— she had never considered this not to be a reasonable arrangement. Being on a disability pension changed her daily life, making it less of an ongoing daily struggle, but challenged her sense of being "legitimate." Negotiating her *specific* body after the departure from the workplace meant reconstituting her identity as "disabled."

The home environment, too, is a site where women with chronic illness re-learn their bodies and environments and move toward structuring their lived spaces as spaces for themselves to be as they are, with chronic illness. Brie's description of her everyday life activities indicates how detailed the disciplining of her environment actually is.

It's as if you say, well, you, even within the house, you cut down the amount of movement you have to make. You know. If I do this, and then this, then I won't have to walk into the other room and back. I remember—it's silly little things—I went down to a seminar in California . . . and I remember thinking—well, I won't take those jeans, because they are buttons and not a zip. See, that's the level of trying to make, it's easier to zip than to button, so that's the state of mind you're in, that you weigh up what the cost of energy [is] per action.

Interviewer: To the tiniest detail almost.

Brie: Well, yeah, because that's the level you live on. . . . Can't do that today. Do that some other time. A few days. Or I would do that—I'd do, say, the [store]. Well, I can't make it to the bank as well. I'll just come home. So, you know, your whole life, you see, because then I have to do like three trips instead of what a person with a car would just do one. Get it all done. Instead you think well, I'll do the bank today, and then in a few days I'll do such a thing, you know? And these years I'm doing no socializing. Or I used to, people sometimes come for tea, but I didn't want to socialize, because it cost me too much. See. An hour or two with people would ruin my day and then I wouldn't shop, couldn't cook. I'd feel terrible. You know? So there's this whole conflict because of course you want to see people, you know, you think you might be OK, but then you're not, and also it's such an effort to think and track what they're saying.

Brie arranges how she uses her time and traverses her space so that she can get done what she needs to without feeling terrible at the end. In order to accommodate her *specific* body, she has re-learned her environment through her body and has re-articulated her body with her environment.

Expressing the specificity of bodies is not site-specific. Women with chronic illness negotiate their *specific* bodies in more than one site. Because of the volatility of bodies, women's negotiations are unpredictable and ever changing. Noreen works two part-time jobs as a counselor; in order to make ends meet, she lives with a roommate and shares her room with her young daughter. She disclosed her illness only to one employer. In both workplaces, her coworkers cover for her when she is not feeling well enough to see clients. Ruth moved to be near a bus stop, bought an electric can opener days after onset of RA, and plans her swimming at the end of her outing so that she does not have to carry the wet suit and towel around for very long. At onset of ME, Elise continually adjusted her paid working schedule from three part-time jobs in counseling to one half-time position in an institutional setting and a small private practice—then to an occasional client with half-time work—then to only the half-time position. She negotiated her paid work environment through a particular constellation of symptoms—cognitive dysfunction and fatigue—trying to create a space of time between meetings and sessions within which she could rebound cognitively. Her choice to take on less paid work and setting limits on interactive communication with clients and coworkers expressed her negotiation of her *specific* body that permitted her to embrace her own volatility and thus resisted *normalization* in a way that set her experience of her ill body in a context that mediated how she could experience paid work while being ill. She bought a new house, tore up the carpets to put in wooden floors, painted with non-toxic paint, and put in a new heating system so that she could live in a chemical-free environment. Her office was de-fumed and re-ventilated as part of detoxifying her working environment. And her intimate spaces with her partner were restructured so that they could explore sexuality while Elise was ill. Through engaging a plethora of social practices, sometimes with other people, these myriad ways women with chronic illness re-link their bodies with their environments and their environments with their bodies show how disciplining the environment radiates out of their own embodiment.

Disciplining the environment by women with chronic illness can be seen as re-patterning the environment to ease movement through social and physical terrains, the matter and the meanings. Ronnie shows how this re-patterning shapes her choices of when and where to be.

I still don't like using a wheelchair, I won't go downtown around noon hour for instance, when I might bump into people I worked with. I don't want to have to deal with that. You know, "Oh what happened to you," kind of thing. I don't want to deal with that. I use it like a car. The car gets me to and from, the wheelchair gets me to and from. It saves my legs so I can go out dancing at night or something, you know, that's how I see it. But other people's perceptions are very negative and I don't like dealing with that shit.

Using a wheelchair for mobility is empowering for Ronnie in the sense that it gets her where she wants to go; however, the social meanings ascribed to the wheelchair are problematic, forcing Ronnie to pattern her activities so that she minimizes negative interaction.

Expressing a *specific* body through re-learning bodies and environments is heightened for women with chronic illness because they are in effect forced to restructure their everyday life in order to accommodate their chronic illness. Many of the women read this as a critical moment to seize, to change their life "for the better." As we mentioned before, many women used spirituality as the basis for "inner healing." Some of these women, as well as other women who did not explicitly refer to spiritual work, framed their experiences of illness as one of learning and listening—"my body is telling me something." Yvonne best expresses this *pharmakon* notion of illness being both a poison and a remedy.

Before I got sick I used to hear a lot of people, or even when I was sick, a lot of people who actually got better from chronic fatigue syndrome, say that it was one of the best things that ever happened to them, was to get sick. Because they found out who they were. They got connected with their bodies again and they found a better way of living. And I didn't understand that for the longest time. And now I am really starting to see the truth in that. Because it was through getting [CFS] that I was able to discover a number of things about myself. One was that I was not connected with my body and any of the feelings in my body, whether they were emotions or sensual feelings or sexuality or not. And that's partly why I got sick, was that I was so disconnected from my body. I wouldn't listen when it got tired or when it got sick or, I just drove over it. When I got sick, it was like my body was saying to me how to reconnect with it.

Yvonne goes on to say that she was living in her head, void of emotion. She desired to reconnect with her body, with her environment in a way that permitted her to be who she was and not who she was supposed to be. Through her "inner work" with a therapist, she realized that she had been sexually abused as a child for a long period of time beginning when she was an infant. She relates the onset of her illness with the inability to no longer suppress those memories because she had driven her physical body so hard.

But with the memories came a lot of gifts because all the emotions and all the
feelings that I had been blocking out, all of those came back. And I had to
learn what I really felt. And who I really was. And part of that, there was a gift
of sexuality came back to me. And I know perhaps a lot of people get sick and
they lose their sexuality, but for me it was the opposite. Before I got sick I was
sexually dead. I had no feeling in my body. I had no idea what a sexual feeling
was. It was like I was literally dead from the waist down. And then getting sick
and having to learn to listen to my body. I'm tired, I'm hungry, this hurts,
this feels good, this doesn't. Having to learn all that, I had no choice any more.
It was either learn or die, basically with the way I was going. I learned to get
in touch with those feelings again, and what an amazing experience it was, if
you can imagine. I learned quite a bit. And one of the most precious gifts I
learned, other than all these feelings and that, was when the sexuality came
back. The big joke was on me because I learned that I wasn't straight, but that
in fact I was gay. And I had no concept of that. And no matter how much I
studied in school and studied feminism, there was the big secret of my life that
I didn't know about. And it was only through getting sick that I was able to
learn all this stuff about myself. So chronic fatigue syndrome has, ironically,
literally been the best thing that has happened in my life so far—bringing
about the truth back to me and starting a healing process on many different
levels.

Yvonne's experience is but one example of how re-learning the body through
chronic illness opens up the possibility of reconstituting identity and re-artic-
ulating with volatile environments. That Yvonne was open to this volatility
encouraged her to reconnect her embodiment with her surrounding environments. Through re-cognition, she was able re-emerge in her corporeal space
as a woman *with* chronic illness.

SPATIALITY AS DISCIPLINING
THE ENVIRONMENT

The structuring of social life through spatiality is a variable process, shifting
with changes in matter and meaning, continually constituting identities,
subjectivities, and bodies. Spatiality as a noun depicts the entirety of social
space, the complete array of social processes comprising any one place, and
the patterns of activities in which people engage, and the physical matter
making up a particular place. Yet because spatiality is a *process*, ceaseless in
its movement, any one configuration—as told through an interview for
example—is but an interim arrangement, having always already been reconstituted prior to being described. Women with chronic illness are in a position to describe how they intervene into processes that produce the complex
texture of social life and restructure their environments so as to accommodate the destabilization of their material body and to redefine what it is for

them to be ill. Their interventions as part of disciplining the environment—sometimes termed adjusting or coping—are at a range of scales: from moving residences to sitting while undertaking meal preparation, from ending intimate relationships to letting the answering machine pick up calls in the evening, and from becoming self-employed to wearing wrist supports while typing. These acts to discipline the environment come about once women with chronic illness have become sensitive to the articulation of constitutive process shaping who she is and how she "fits" in her immediate surroundings. If women with chronic illness are embedded within a web of social relations imbued with power and draw on their own embodiment as a source of knowledge to frame their activities, then what are the implications of being chronically ill for spatiality?

We suggest that women with chronic illness restructure social and physical environments by re-learning environments through chronically ill bodies. After onset of illness, a woman with chronic illness reconstitutes her identity by re-learning who she is *with chronic illness* and how she is re-placed, re-positioned, and re-embedded in social relations of power of a particular deployment of power/knowledge/space. As each woman re-learns her body—discursively and materially—she redefines illness, reconnects with matter and meaning, and re-emerges as a *specific* body.

10

Connections

Lying flat. At last. . . . Hum. . . . I'm so tired. Maybe I'll be able to sleep through the night. Maybe I shouldn't have taken that nap this afternoon. I wonder how much napping affects sleeping. On the weekends, I only do the bare minimum and nap on and off all day. And don't sleep. Even on my long days, I don't sleep . . . it probably doesn't matter. "No thanks. I don't need any water." *. . . Okay, if I can just settle down. I should probably do a few more sets of exercises. . . . No. I'm too tired. Just relax. . . . What was that exercise to make you go to sleep? Which book was it in? Let me just get it. . . . Page 73. . . . Relax all body parts. Sequence. Concentrate on feeling limp. I remember now. Okay. . . . Toes. Tingling. Ankles. Knees. Thighs. Ouch. Still hurts. Relax. Hands. Elbows. Stomach. Chest. Shoulders. Neck. . . . Yes, . . . this feels better. . . . Now, go to sleep. . . . Relax. . . .* "Good night, honey. I love you, too." *I've got to do this again. Relax. . . . Toes . . . ankles . . . hands . . . neck. . . . This isn't working. . . . Start again. . . . Relax. . . . Feet . . . ankles . . . knees. . . . The doctor! Tomorrow. Tomorrow's Wednesday. Yes, at 2:30. I remember looking it up. Would it be better to have my short day on Wednesdays? Just for recovery. Maybe not. I'm so exhausted now. Oh my gosh! What am I like on Thursdays? I don't think I know. Maybe I won't think about that right now. . . . Relax. . . . If I knew what to do, my body would be different. No, my body wouldn't be different. I would be different. I would know what to do, which medicines to take, how much to exercise. Tomorrow, I'll know. . . . Well, perhaps not everything, but I'll know something. . . . The laundry, I forgot to do the laundry. . . . Something that should help me . . . in some way . . . I don't want to be sick anymore.*

TOWARD A RADICAL BODY POLITICS

We set out for a goal of this book an exposition of a feminist materialist analytical framework for understanding and explaining the body. The body

165

we used to illustrate our arguments was the body with chronic illness, as accessed through 49 women's accounts of living with Myalgic Encephalomyelitis (ME) and Rheumatoid Arthritis (RA). Feminist explanations of bodies that interested us generally focused on how power influences the constitution of the self, subjectivity, and identity. We argued that, inevitably, the social and the spatial are steeped together, inextricably linked, caught up in the other, forever reproducing themselves. Within this context, thinking through the body with chronic illness as indeterminable opened up ways to understand the body as both discursive and material at the same time. Wanting to capture the uncertainty of everyday life socially, spatially, financially, and bodily, we used the concepts *"bodies in context," corporeal space,* and *embodiment* to describe the constitutive processes of self and identity as well as of environment, experience, and embeddedness. Our efforts found that being in a state of flux constituted the parameters of women's environments as permeable borders, expanding and contracting in relation to the disease process, the physicality of the home and workplace, and meanings of illness ascribed to a body with chronic illness. Social relations of power, too, placed the women in a larger context, bringing to bear collectively the close relationship they had with the environments they traversed daily. The milieus within and through which women with chronic illness lived their daily lives were situated within the dominant configuration of the deployment of power as expressed in Victoria and Vancouver, British Columbia, in the mid- to late-1990s.

Because of the way we framed our arguments in this book, this is a historically specific analysis. We focused on the nexus of women, body, illness—the devalued sides of the binaries with men, thought, and health, hoping to loosen the tight hold these binaries have in shaping much theoretical thinking about women's ill bodies. In loosening these seemingly resolute bindings, we can perhaps understand better how the expression of competing identities—ill, healthy, abled, disabled, not ill, not healthy, not abled, and not disabled—can exist for one woman, at one time, in one environment at the same time. When working with these identities, a new politics opens up, one that is based on *specific* bodies in *specific* environments. Embracing the volatility of bodies in a politics of everyday life makes possible the emergence of self as a continual process, especially in relation to "bodies in context," with an ongoing negotiation of identity expressions. The synchronous notion of bodily being as discursive and material facilitates an understanding of how the social and the spatial constitute self and identity in that the specificity of a body with chronic illness emerges from the messy world of everyday living and not as a naturalized ill body (either because of a diagnosis or a disease process) in need of discipline (through various mechanisms developed through power/knowledge/space to sustain dominance). Rather, an unstable politics surfaces that is articulated through a specific intersection of temporary identities (a nodal point), that can be just as fleeting, ephemeral, and fragile as any one identity. This momentary solidification of a collective identity can be a departure point to effect change.

A central feature of this radical body politics is the conceptualization of discourse and materiality, not as a dualism, but as ways to draw attention to bodily variation as a state of being. Refusing to break living connections and focusing on the "mass of mess" integral to bodily experience is not as restrictive analytically as seductively sorting the body into categories for conceptual ease. Relaxing the hold of binary thinking reveals discursive and material fissures wide enough to read the body differently. In reading the body differently, conventional topics associated with the body, such as experience, can be reconceived and rethought in the context of spatiality. If "experience is an interpretation and in need of interpretation,"[1] then "troubling" experience, including the sensorial and emotional, has to be part of understanding the body. If not, the specificity of bodies and environments would be lost because the notion of constitution would fall flat, producing only uniform identities and space based on "likeness" and "unity." But we know this not to be the case. Environments, like identities, also become *specific*, textured in everyday life, holding some material form through temporarily fixed capital. Spatiality as a constitutive process is as in flux and as fleeting as expressions of individual and collective identities; with its temporal and spatial fixity, an intersection of a specific deployment of power/knowledge/space at any given point in time. Connecting spatiality with "troubling" experience means that we can scrutinize the circumstances within and through which a series of acts, or sets of bodily activities, constitute themselves as a bodily experience—discursively or materially.

DEMONSTRATING THEORY

Our approach to presenting our exposition of a radical body politics in this book took the form of demonstrating theory through accounts of women's experiences of chronic illness. The analysis was neither theory-driven nor empirically derived. Rather, the analysis wove together our thoughts about body and space and our readings of the information about everyday life provided to us by women with chronic illness. The tightness with which we braided our own concepts with the women's accounts was intended to be uneven. This unevenness permits us to maintain our commitment to providing analytical space to assess critically our own ideas of "making sense" of chronic illness. Underlying our argument has been the notion that understanding knowledge, just as understanding bodies, identities, and environments, arises from the messy world of everyday life. Yet to claim that understanding can only arise from the mundane or from experience diminishes the significance that thinking about understanding can have in explaining the mundane and experience. Our advocacy of "troubling" experience helps to prevent us from falling into the trap of claiming that drawing theory from experience is inherently liberating. We know that any discourse can be dangerous in the sense that any discourse can sustain dominance by normalizing bodily ideals and bodily activities (as part of self-formation) to the detriment of women's capacities to resist and transform social relations of power. Going back and forth between theory and data was an especially effective way for us to maneuver through the binary of discourse and materiality and the fluctuations of bodies, identities, and environments.

What this uneven weaving of concepts and accounts of experiences means is that a systematic application of concepts is lacking. As well, examples demonstrating theoretical points can appear trite. For example, "*pharmakon*" is a deceptively simple concept. Meaning both medicine and poison, *pharmakon* can illustrate the simultaneity of being located in oppositional states of being at the same time. We used this notion to draw out the experience of illness as being both negative and positive, restrictive and liberating, and debilitating and healing (see chapter 9). However, the complexity of the various ways in which illness can be both devastating and rejuvenating is quashed in favor of promoting the argument of illness initiates a process whereby women with chronic illness re-learn the environment through the fluctuating destabilization of their body materially and discursively. This is not to say that we would not recognize the importance of elaborating the complexity of *pharmakon*; rather, we use the concept of *pharmakon* in its complexity to make our point about re-learning environments.

Similar arguments can be made about the invocation of other concepts we have used in our radical body politics such as the constitutive outside, nodal point, power/knowledge/space, corporeal space, embodiment, and "bodies in context." But it is through our use of these concepts that we have been able to unsettle dualisms, especially those associated with discourse and materiality, opening up analytical spaces to assist in understanding body, identity, and space. We, in turn, flood these spaces with notions of tension, in betweenness, filtering, and transition as we attempt to make sense of the bodies, experiences, and environments of women with chronic illness. For example, we have defined inscription as a process of discursive and material practices through which a particular rendering of an idealized or fleshed body is etched onto a body (see chapter 6). Implicit in the conceptualization of inscription as a process, is that inscription does not take place in a vacuum on pre-discursive or pre-mattered bodies. Inscription applies to bodies already embedded in social relations of power that are already located in the dominant configuration of a specific deployment of power/knowledge/space. It is through these sets of relations that inscription works to discipline, regulate, normalize, and naturalize particular bodies. Being able to decipher power in this context permits someone to trace these bodily "markings" and make them culturally intelligible. Thus, in conceiving inscription as a process, we are able to show how women's experiences of diagnosis, for example, filter an idealized body with a fleshed one. Women's accounts of their experiences of diagnoses highlight the transition from a relatively stable material body to one that was uncertain in its destabilization. Making sense of this filtering for the women meant holding the two in tension so that they could negotiate their identity as either both healthy and ill, or somewhere in between.

THREE MORE TENSIONS

In our demonstration of our exposition of a radical body politics, three sets of tensions emerged as we tried to "fit" our analysis with our own worldviews. First is the tension between individual and collective accounts of experience. Our focus on the body is not the same as heightening the notion of the individual. It may appear that our intense scrutiny of the body through individual examples of experience eclipses any collectivity that women with chronic illness might have for a collective politics. The radical body politics proposed here is not solely about individual women's bodies and how women cope with illness; rather, this framework permits insight into the processes through which women experience illness, shape their notions of "self," express identities, and structure their environments. Through this insight, there can be a collective politics. Women do not exist in isolation to each other or to anyone else. The notion of context and corporeal space through what can be termed a "microgeography of embodiment" permits a collective way to look at individual bodies. Through reframing body politics along these lines, the future for women's bodies remains radical and open to numerous possibilities—ones which can assist women in overcoming the ways power is deployed without reinforcing them.

Second is the tension between political economic and poststructural accounts of the organization of the social relations of power. Our use of poststructural insights is not the same as a poststructural analysis of women's accounts of chronic illness. It may appear that our account does not adequately attend to the women's class locations. Our understanding of labor, labor processes, and class location is closely aligned with feminist accounts of political economy.[2] Yet we find useful poststructural and post-Marxist concepts in making sense of bodies and space because they help us to understand aspects of life that do not easily "fit" into conventional political economy at the scale we want to understand them—as experiences of everyday life. We know that most women do not have the means nor the access to resources to do as Barbara did and hire a nanny for childcare or as Elise did and buy and renovate a house to accommodate chronic illness. This is not the case for most women, period. But our point in citing these examples was not to offer these as *the* path for disciplining the social and physical environment to accommodate chronic illness; rather, our point was to illustrate how *some women* attempt to restructure their environments so as to coordinate more closely their lived spaces (embodiment) with their social and physical environments.

Third is the tension among the multiple facets of embeddedness in the social relations of power. Our concentration on women's experiences of chronic illness is not the same as privileging women, experience, or chronic illness in analysis. It may appear that we ignored privilege theoretically when we drew only on these particular women's experiences empirically. We recognize that while intersections, for example, of citizenship, ethnicity, race, and sexuality with gender were not prominent in this study, bodies are inscribed by the multiple discourses linked to such social locations. Clearly, from our discussion, we would expect other discourses, from other places and from other cultures, to mediate how ill bodies are made culturally intelligible and are lived.[3] Further, women located at these intersections within Canada, where this study took place, may have had an additional or different empirical specificity to day-to-day issues, although we would anticipate and intend our concepts to have further theoretical reach than the "particular" as presented here. We did not seek to problematize any social location other than ability, as expressed in terms of chronic illness, in developing a radical body politics. This does not mean that privilege was ignored. Privilege was integral to the women's experiences. We happened to cast this partly as implicated in discourse, partly in materiality, partly in identity, and partly in spatiality. Our approach to recruitment signals the primary reason for having only white women with Canadian citizenship with European ethnic backgrounds in the study.[4] The choice to access women diagnosed with ME or RA through support groups and other community networks constituted the parameters within which we accessed potential study participants. We know that women of color, that non-citizens,[5] and that women from ethnic backgrounds other than those represented by the women in this study were part of these support groups and social networks, but none answered the recruitment flyer. Accessing *specific* women's bodies according to social location would need to have involved active selection.

PATIENCE AND WOMEN LIKE HER

In relation to this framework, it does not matter whether Patience is diagnosed with a chronic illness tomorrow, next week, or next year. Making sense of her experiences is what is at issue. In scrutinizing accounts of women's experiences of chronic illness, we have tried to show how crucial an understanding of women's embodiment in their corporeal spaces and as "bodies in context" is in being able to articulate a reconstituted self, express fluctuating identities, and restructure social and physical environments. Women with chronic illness are involved in a variety of discursive and material practices—some imposed, such as diagnosis, others self-forming, such as bodily activities—that define what it is to be ill. These definitions, made culturally intelligible through the etchings inscribed onto an ill body, are used by the women themselves, their friends and family, insurance companies, and employers to determine the legitimacy of a woman's claim to be ill. These inscriptions are incomplete and contradictory, forming borders that are thus permeable, fluctuating, and fluid, leaving space for competing readings of ill bodies. Because they exist within these borders of illness, women are able to resist dominant readings of ill bodies, and engage in practices that redefine the parameters through which their own bodies can be defined. There are material limits—physiologically, anatomically, financially—which constrain women's choices and actions. Within these milieus, women's subjectivities are reconstituted and "new" selves emerge. In living their environments through embodiment, women are able to access points around which to "fix," at least temporarily, an "ill" identity without naturalizing it as "lack of health." Women engage in disciplining the environment, predicated upon the notion of volatility, so that their temporary identities can assist in organizing bodily activities in ways that undermine hegemony and challenge the prevailing deployment of power/knowledge/space.

In relation to her experience of chronic illness, it does matter that Patience has chronic illness and does not want to be sick anymore. "Not being sick anymore" entails not wanting the physical sensation of pain, fatigue, forgetfulness, nausea, dizziness, and foggy thinking as well as not wanting to be inscribed by either an idealized healthy body or fleshed ill one. Embracing the volatility of an ill body is not easy; it is merely a way to rethink the ill body so that having chronic illness is no longer marginalizing biomedically, socially, or economically. Having chronic illness could be just another way to be.

Notes

NOTES FOR CHAPTER 1

1. See, for example, Isabel Dyck, "Hidden Geographies: The Changing Life-worlds of Women with Disabilities," *Social Science and Medicine* 40 (1995): 307–20; Pamela Moss, "Negotiating Spaces in Home Environments: Older Women Living with Arthritis," *Social Science and Medicine* 45 (1997): 23–33; Isabel Dyck, "Women with Disabilities and Everyday Geographies: Home Space and the Contested Body," in *Putting Health into Place: Landscape, Identity and Wellbeing*, ed. Robin A. Kearns and Wil Gesler (Syracuse, N.Y.: Syracuse Press, 1998), 102–9; Isabel Dyck, "Body Troubles: Women, the Workplace, and Negotiations of a Disabled Identity," in *Mind and Body Spaces: Geographies of Illness, Impairment, and Disability*, ed. Ruth Butler and Hester Parr (New York: Routledge, 1999), 119–37; Pamela Moss and Isabel Dyck, "Journeying through ME: Identity, the Body, and Women with Chronic Illness," in *Embodied Geographies: Spaces, Bodies and Rites of Passage*, ed. Elizabeth Kenworthy Teather (New York: Routledge, 1999), 157–74; Pamela Moss and Isabel Dyck, "Material Bodies Precariously Positioned: Working Women Diagnosed with Chronic Illness," in *Geographies of Women's Health*, ed. Isabel Dyck, Nancy Davis Lewis, and Sara McLafferty (New York: Routledge, 2001), 231–47. Although we have published research papers arising out of the project we work with here, this book is not a collection of those works or a recycling of those ideas. Rather, the book is an extended analysis of some of the ideas we have briefly taken up in some of the articles. For example, in Pamela Moss and Isabel Dyck, "Inquiry into Environment and Body: Women, Work and Chronic Illness," *Environment & Planning D: Society & Space* 14 (1996): 737–53, we introduce basic ideas for the framework we propose in this book. Similarly, in Pamela Moss and Isabel Dyck, "Body, Corporeal Space, and Legitimating Chronic Illness: Women Diagnosed with ME," *Antipode* 31 (1999): 372–97, we introduce the concept of *corporeal space*, which is one aspect of the framework described in chapter 4.

2. On sexuality, see, for example, David Bell and Gill Valentine, eds., *Maps of Desire* (New York: Routledge, 1995). On various aspects of the constitution of bodies and space, see, for example, Nancy Duncan, ed., *Body/Space: Destabilizing Geographies of Gender and Sexuality* (New York: Routledge, 1996). On multiple ways the

body manifests in particular places, see, for example, Heidi J. Nast and Steve Pile, eds., *Places through the Body* (New York: Routledge, 1998). On medicalized spaces, see, for example, Hester Parr and Chris Philo, "Mapping 'Mad' Identities," in *Mapping the Subject: Geographies of Cultural Transformation*, ed. Steve Pile and Nigel Thrift (New York: Routledge, 1995), 199–225. On physical space, see, for example, Ruth Butler and Sophie Bowlby, "Disabled Bodies in Public Space," *Environment & Planning D: Society & Space* 15 (1997): 411–33.

3. In addition to Nast and Pile, *Places through the Body*, two other collections of such work include Ruth Butler and Hester Parr, eds., *Mind and Body Spaces: Geographies of Illness, Impairment, and Disability* and Elizabeth Kenworthy Teather, ed., *Embodied Geographies: Spaces, Bodies and Rites of Passage*.

4. See Michel Foucault, *History of Sexuality, Volume 1: An Introduction* (New York: Vintage, 1978) and *Discipline and Punish: The Birth of the Prison* (New York: Vintage, 1979). For exemplars of French feminist psychoanalysis, see for example Hélène Cixous, "Castration or Decapitation?" *Signs* 7 (1981), 41–55; Julia Kristeva, *Revolution in Poetic Language*, trans. Margaret Walker (New York: Columbia University Press, 1984); Julia Kristeva, *Tales of Love*, trans. Leon S. Roudiez (New York: Columbia University Press, 1987); and Hélène Cixous and Catherine Clément, *The Newly Born Woman*, trans. Betsy Wing (Minneapolis: University of Minnesota Press, 1986).

5. Judith Butler, *Gender Trouble: Feminism and the Subversion of Identity* (New York: Routledge, 1990) and *Bodies That Matter: On the Discursive Limits of "Sex"* (New York: Routledge, 1993).

6. Susan Bordo, *Unbearable Weight: Feminism, Western Culture, and the Body* (Berkeley: University of California Press, 1993) and Moira Gatens, *Imaginary Bodies* (New York: Routledge, 1996).

7. Elizabeth Grosz, *Volatile Bodies: Toward a Corporeal Feminism* (Bloomington: Indiana University Press, 1994).

8. Nona Y. Glazer, "Servants to Capital: Unpaid Domestic Labor and Paid Work," *Review of Radical Political Economics* 16, no. 1 (1984): 61–87.

9. Mary O'Brien, *The Politics of Reproduction* (London: Routledge & Kegan Paul, 1981).

10. Felicity J. Callard, "The Body in Theory," *Environment & Planning: Society & Space* 16 (1998): 387–400.

11. See, for example, Linda McDowell, "Towards an Understanding of the Gender Division of Urban Space," *Environment and Planning D; Society and Space* 1 (1983), 15–30; Doreen Massey, *Spatial Divisions of Labour* (London: Macmillan, 1984); Geraldine Pratt, "Reflections on Poststructuralism and Feminist Empirics," *Antipode* 25 (1993): 51–63; Gillian Rose, *Feminism and Geography: The Limits of Geographical Knowledge* (Minneapolis: University of Minneisota Press, 1993); Vera Chouinard and Ali Grant, "On Not Being Anywhere Near the 'Project,'" *Antipode* 27 (1995): 137–66; and Julie-Kathy Gibson-Graham, *The End of Capitalism (As We Knew It): A Feminist Critique of Political Economy* (Oxford: Blackwell, 1996).

12. See, for example, the collection by Michael Keith and Steve Pile, eds., *Place and the Politics of Identity* (New York: Routledge, 1993), in particular see Liz Bondi, "Locating Identity Politics," 84–101. In another interesting, though not explicitly

feminist, work, Wolfgang Natter and John Paul Jones III, in "Identity, Space and Other Uncertainties," in *Space and Social Theory: Interpreting Modernity and Postmodernity*, ed. Georges Benko and Ulf Strohmayer (Oxford: Blackwell, 1997), 141–61, argue for nonessential identities and spaces such that room is opened up for practicing uncertainties. And Linda McDowell and Gill Court, in "Performing Work: Bodily Representations in Merchant Banks," *Environment and Planning D: Society and Space* 12 (1994): 727–50, show how certain bodies act out their jobs in specific places.

13. John Paul Jones III, Heidi J. Nast, and Susan M. Roberts, eds., *Thresholds in Feminist Geography: Difference, Methodology, Representation* (Lanham, Md.: Rowman & Littlefield, 1997).

14. The exchange between Andrea Litva and John Eyles, "Coming Out: Exposing Social Theory in Medical Geography," *Health & Place* 1 (1995): 5–14, and Chris Philo, "Staying In? Invited Comments on 'Coming Out': Exposing Social Theory in Medical Geography," *Health & Place* 2 (1996): 35–40, highlights some of the lacunae in the literature in health geography. The sole focus on women in *Geographies of Women's Health*, ed. Isabel Dyck, Nancy Davis Lewis, and Sara McLafferty (New York: Routledge, 2001) is encouraging, especially the four chapters devoted to women's bodies: Joyce Davidson, "Fear and Trembling in the Mall: Women, Agoraphobia, and Body Boundaries," 213–30; Andrea Litva, Kay Peggs, and Graham Moon, "The Beauty of Health: Locating Young Women's Health and Appearance," 248–64; Pamela Moss and Isabel Dyck, "Material Bodies Precariously Positioned: Women Embodying Chronic Illness in the Workplace," 231–47; and Yvonne Underhill-Sem, " 'The Baby Is Turning': Child-bearing in Wanigela, Oro Province, Papua New Guinea," 197–212.

For examples outside of health geography, see David Bell, Jon Binnie, Julia Cream, and Gill Valentine, "All Hyped Up and No Place to Go," *Gender, Place & Culture* 1 (1994): 31–48; Julia Cream, "Women on Trial? A Private Pillory?" in *Mapping the Subject: Geographies of Cultural Transformation*, 158–69; Robyn Longhurst and Lynda Johnston, "Embodying Places and Emplacing Bodies: Pregnant Women and Women Body Builders," in *Feminist Thought in Aotearoa/New Zealand*, ed. Rosemary DuPlessis and Lynne Alice (Auckland, N.Z.: Oxford University Press 1998), 156–63; and Geraldine Pratt, in collaboration with the Philippine Women Centre, Vancouver, Canada, "Inscribing Domestic Work on Filipina Bodies," in *Places through the Body*, 283–304.

15. The future of health geography has been addressed by John Eyles, "From Disease Ecology and Spatial Analysis To . . . ? The Challenges of Medical Geography in Canada," *Health and Canadian Society* 1 (1993): 113–45, and Robin Kearns and Alun E. Joseph, "Space in Its Place: Developing the Link in Medical Geography," *Social Science and Medicine* 37 (1993): 711–17, both of which identify the need for critical perspectives.

16. Michael Dorn and Glenda Laws, "Social Theory, Body Politics, and Medical Geography: Extending Kearns's Invitation," *The Professional Geographer* 46 (1994): 106–10.

17. In addition to Hester Parr and Chris Philo, "Mapping 'Mad' Identities," see Michael Dorn, "Beyond Nomadism: The Travel Narratives of a 'Cripple,' " in *Places*

through the Body, 183–206. A collection of disability works is reviewed in Deborah C. Park, John P. Radford, and Michael H. Vickers, "Disability Studies in Human Geography," *Progress in Human Geography* 22 (1998): 208–33.

18. One of the strongest proponents of the social disability model is Mike Oliver, *Understanding Disability: From Theory to Practice* (Basingstoke, U.K.: Macmillan, 1996). In geography, for example, see Brendan Gleeson, *Geographies of Disability* (New York: Routledge, 1999); Rob F. Imrie, *Disability and the City: International Perspectives* (London: Paul Chapmen, 1996); and Ruth Butler and Sophia Bowlby, "Bodies and Spaces: An Exploration of Disabled People's Experiences of Public Space," *Environment and Planning D: Society and Space* 15 (1997): 411–33. The absence of the body in much of this research is also noted by Edward Hall in " 'Blood, Brain and Bones': Taking the Body Seriously in the Geography of Health and Impairment," *Area* 32 (2000): 21–30.

19. Genevieve Lloyd, *The Man of Reason: 'Male' and 'Female' in Western Philosophy* (Minneapolis: University of Minnesota Press, 1984). Linda J. Nicholson, ed., *Feminism/Postmodernism* (New York: Routledge, 1990) has become a classic as an introduction to the tension between feminism and postmodernism.

20. Jacques Derrida, "Plato's Pharmacy," in *Dissemination*, trans. Barbara Johnson (Chicago: University of Chicago Press, 1981), 61–172. For definitions of *pharmakon* in this brief discussion, see especially pages 70–71 and 120. Derrida also uses the concept of *pharmakon* as perfume: as a cosmetic to conceal its own death under the veil of the living, to hide itself as it is (142).

21. Many of Chantal Mouffe's works contain descriptions of the ways she uses the "constitutive outside." Ones that we find most useful are "Post-Marxism: Democracy and Identity," *Environment & Planning D: Society and Space* 13 (1995): 259–65 and "Feminism, Citizenship and Radical Democratic Politics," in *Feminists Theorize the Political*, ed. Judith Butler and Joan W. Scott (New York: Routledge, 1992), 369–84.

22. Elizabeth Grosz, in *Space, Time, and Perversion* (New York: Routledge, 1995), a philosopher, explores how her ideas about corporeality, sexuality, and space articulate with and possibly contaminate concepts from architecture, geography, and physics. As a geographer, Nancy Duncan, in *Body/Space*, includes works that adhere to the idea that bodies constitute and are constituted through space and that gender and sexuality are part of the material context of spaces and places. Rosa Ainley, *New Frontiers of Space, Bodies and Gender* (New York: Routledge, 1998), a photojournalist, pulls together a collection of feminist works on space that show how space is just not a place where activities take place; rather, space is something that shapes and is shaped by the ways in which we actually *do* gender.

23. In addition to the works mentioned in the previous note, see Doreen Massey, *Space, Place, and Gender* (Minneapolis: University of Minnesota Press, 1995), in particular, "A Global Sense of Place," 146–56, and Edward W. Soja, *Thirdspace: Journeys to Los Angeles and Other Real-and-Imagined Places* (Oxford: Blackwell, 1996).

24. Pamela Moss and Isabel Dyck, "Inquiry into Environment and Body," 744. See also Pamela Moss and Isabel Dyck, "Body, Corporeal Space, and Legitimating Chronic Illness," 377.

25. Ruth Pinder, "Sick-but-fit or Fit-but-sick? Ambiguity and Identity in the Workplace," in *Exploring the Divide: Illness and Disability*, ed. Colin Barnes and Geoff Mercer (Leeds: Disability Press, 1996), 135–56.

26. bell hooks, "Choosing the Margin as a Space of Radical Openness," in *Yearning: Race, Gender, and Cultural Politics* (Boston: South End Press, 1990), reprinted in *Women, Knowledge, and Reality*, ed. Ann Garry and Marilyn Pearsall (New York: Routledge, 1996), 48–55.

27. Whether or not the body would still be marked with shackles of ignominy, abjection, or deviance is a theme we take up in chapter 8.

NOTES FOR CHAPTER 2

1. Susan Bordo, *Unbearable Weight: Feminism, Western Culture, and the Body* (Berkeley: University of California Press, 1993); Rosalyn Diprose, *The Bodies of Women: Ethics, Embodiment, and Sexual Difference* (New York: Routledge, 1993); Moira Gatens, *Imaginary Bodies* (New York: Routledge, 1996); Elizabeth Grosz, *Volatile Bodies: Toward a Corporeal Feminism* (Bloomington: Indiana University Press, 1994); Emily Martin, *Flexible Bodies: The Role of Immunity in American Culture from the Days of Polio to the Age of AIDS* (Boston: Beacon Press, 1994); Kathy Davis, *Reshaping the Female Body: The Dilemma of Cosmetic Surgery* (New York: Routledge, 1995); and Margrit Shildrick, *Leaky Bodies and Boundaries: Feminism, Postmodernism and (Bio)Ethics* (New York: Routledge, 1997).

2. Alongside articles scattered throughout various journals (which we discuss later), many of these geographical works on the body have appeared as collections of articles, most of which were introduced in chapter 1. But this is not always the case. See, for example, Alison Blunt and Jane Wills, "Embodying Geography: Feminist Geographies of Gender," in *Dissident Geographies: An Introduction to Radical Ideas and Practice* (Harlow: Longman, 2000), 90–127 and Linda McDowell, "In and Out of Place: Bodies and Embodiment," in *Gender, Identity, and Place: Understanding Feminist Geographies* (Oxford: Polity Press, 1999), 34–70.

3. There is no doubt that the "perfect body" is racialized white. See discussions in Lee Monaghan, "Creating 'The Perfect Body': A Variable Project," *Body & Society* 5, nos. 2 and 3 (1999): 267–90; and Karla Henderson and Barbara Ainsworth, "Researching Leisure and Physical Activity with Women of Color: Issues and Emerging Questions," *Leisure Sciences* 23, no. 1 (2001): 21–34.

4. There is also no doubt that the "perfect body" is also abled. See Sharon Dale Stone, "The Myth of Bodily Perfection," *Disability and Society* 10 (1995): 413–24.

5. Lynda Johnston, "The Politics of the Pump: Hard Core Gyms and Women Body Builders," *New Zealand Geographer* 15, no. 3 (1995): 16–18 and "Flexing Femininity: Female Body Builders Refiguring 'The Body,'" *Gender, Place, and Culture* 3 (1996): 327–40, worked with female body builders to get a sense of how popular "beautiful" body images might be linked to changes in women's physical bodies. In her work, she contrasts the rather negative image of female body builders as ugly, muscular, and masculine with the more subversive image of a female body builder as sexy, trim, and beautiful. She found that women were relatively keen to

show off their bodies—as "success" stories—and knowingly set themselves up for a public(ized) consumptive gaze as part of the process of defining themselves as beautiful, confident, and sexy. This drive for what we would call "successful beauty" is especially enhanced when celebrities make the case. White female celebrities regularly promote beauty products—Andie McDowell with make-up, Sarah Jessica Parker with hair color, and Kate Moss with perfume. Other celebrities promote fitness through carefully developed aerobic fitness routines for women at all ages—Angela Lansbury, Jane Fonda, Elle MacPherson, Carnie Wilson, Marla Maples, and Kathy Ireland. Cher developed her video set after her recovery from Myalgic Encephalomyelitis. Some celebrities do not have to produce and star in videos to popularize a path to fitness and well-being. For example, Madonna popularized Ashtanga Yoga as a way to blend spiritual awareness with body fitness. Ashtanga, a vigorous practice composed of three sequences—*Yoga Chikitsa, Nadi Shodhana, Sthira Bhaga*—that align, purify, and strengthen the eight systems of the body, is one of the most effective types of yoga for toning, building muscles, and maintaining cardiovascular health. The result, for Madonna at least, is a "beautiful" body and a balanced sense of self, psychologically and spiritually. For the consuming "eye," Madonna still "fits" the notion of "successful beauty," even after giving birth to two children.

6. Feminist bioethics is a growing field of study. Rosemarie Tong, *Feminist Approaches to Bioethics: Theoretical Reflections and Practical Applications* (Boulder, Colo.: Westview, 1997) provides a good overview of the field. Other works that have influenced our thinking include Rosalyn Diprose, *The Bodies of Women*; Margrit Shildrick, *Leaky Bodies and Boundaries*; and Anne Donchin and Laura Martha Purdy, *Embodying Bioethics: Recent Feminist Advances* (Lanham, Md.: Rowman & Littlefield, 1999).

7. Lee Edelman, "The Plague of Discourse: Politics, Literary Theory, and AIDS," in *The Postmodern Turn: New Perspectives on Social Theory*, ed. Steven Seidman (Cambridge: Cambridge University Press, 1994), 299–312, writes about the inability to separate AIDS as a disease from its representations, to separate the literal from the figurative. Reading Edelman's work, we are struck by how important it is to maintain bodies with AIDS and bodies infected with HIV within the discourse, for with an excision of such bodies, the project of reading discourse is no longer political.

8. Elaine Showalter, *Hystories: Hysterical Epidemics and Modern Media* (New York: Columbia University Press, 1997) includes arguments about collective cultural anxiety at the turn of the century over bodily manifestations of fin-de-siècle angst. Activists involved with recovered memory syndrome and Gulf War Syndrome spoke out against Showalter's claim that cultural anxiety takes the form of hysterical moments in history. Showalter's notion of how cultural angst expresses itself through illness has been challenged analytically by people studying Chronic Fatigue Syndrome. Lesley Cooper and Martin Walker, "Whose Hysteria?" *Continuum* 5, no. 1 (1997): 4–5; and Peggy Munson, "The Paradox of Lost Fingerprints: Metaphor and the Shaming of Chronic Fatigue Syndrome," in *Stricken: Voices from the Hidden Epidemic of Chronic Fatigue Syndrome*, ed. Peggy Munson (New York: Haworth, 2000), 95–126, provide critical responses to Showalter's thesis. Cooper and Walker argue that the "hysteria theory" de-legitimizes the experiences of people with

Chronic Fatigue Syndrome and forces treatment into the realm of psychiatry. This movement into psychiatry, and consequently science and medicine, prohibits people with Chronic Fatigue Syndrome from participating in the construction of the discourse of the illness. Munson takes a different path of criticism and argues that Showalter undertook "bad" research and did not look at any of the medical literature that clearly shows Chronic Fatigue Syndrome is a disease of the body, not of the mind. She supports her argument by quoting physicians' responses to Showalter's work and by showing how easily dismissed individual experiences of Chronic Fatigue Syndrome are in the media through, for example, televised interviews and debates. Although we do not think that all collective anxiety can be defined as hysterical moments, we do think that there are collective manifestations of cultural angst. One such form in popular media points simultaneously to the limits and possibilities of bodies and their bodily forms, and as Cooper and Walker argue, discourses of psychiatry, science, and medicine, and we would add media, are significant in the role of defining illness and creating cultural angst. Ironically, although giving too much authority to the discourses of biomedicine, Munson demonstrates more clearly the point Showalter was trying to make: media plays a prominent role in the social construction of collective views of illness.

9. See Elspeth Probyn, *Sexing the Self: Gendered Positions in Cultural Studies* (New York: Routledge, 1993); Butler, *Gender Trouble: Feminism and the Subversion of Identity* (New York: Routledge, 1990); Angela Davis, *Women, Race, and Class* (New York: Random House, 1981); and Nancy K. Miller, *Getting Personal: Feminist Occasions and Other Autobiographical Acts* (New York: Routledge, 1993).

10. Rereading classical sociological texts, both Simon J. Williams and Gillian A. Bendelow, "Sociology and the 'Problem' of the Body," in *The Lived Body: Sociological Themes, Embodied Issues* (New York: Routledge, 1998), 9–24; and David Harvey, "The Body as an Accumulation Strategy," *Environment & Planning D: Society & Space* 16 (1999): 401–21, reinsinuate the body as part of the modern project. Williams and Bendelow, as we argue below, focus on unsettling dualistic thinking, whereas Harvey demonstrates that Marx's underlying theory of body formation can assist in understanding how people engage in a politics that challenges the conditions under which they labor.

11. By "counterhegemonic circles," we are referring to groups of persons who collectively adhere to notions seemingly alternative to the hegemony. To illustrate this point further, even within say hippie or "granola" lifestyles, there are "prescriptive" bodily notions that are part of concrete social practices that assist in creating an image specific to that group.

12. Anne Witz, "Whose Body Matters? Feminist Sociology and the Corporeal Turn in Sociology and Feminism," *Body and Society* 6, no. 2 (2000): 1–24.

13. Chris Shilling, *The Body and Social Theory* (Thousand Oaks, Calif.: Sage, 1993), 41–99.

14. Elizabeth Grosz, *Volatile Bodies,* 32, emphasis in original.

15. It used to be legal in Canada to introduce a sexual assault victim's sexual history into court, including rape cases, if it assisted in the defense of the accused perpetrator.

16. Elizabeth Grosz, *Volatile Bodies,* 38.

17. Simon J. Williams and Gillian A. Bendelow, *The Lived Body*, 9–66.

18. For their discussion of "order," they draw on works such as Robert Hertz, *Death and the Right Hand* (New York: Cohen and West, 1960 [1909]); Mary Douglas, *Natural Symbols: Explorations in Cosmology* (London: Cresset Press, 1970); Norbert Elias, *The Civilizing Process, Volume 2: State Formation and Civilization* (Oxford: Basil Blackwell, 1982 [1939]); Michel Foucault, *The Birth of a Clinic: An Archaeology of Medical Perception* (New York: Vintage, 1973); and Bryan S. Turner, *The Body and Society*, 2nd ed. (Oxford: Basil Blackwell, 1996).

19. For their discussion of "control," they draw on works like Marcel Mauss, "Techniques of the Body," *Economy and Society* 2 (1973 [1934]): 70–88; Maurice Merleau-Ponty, *The Phenomenology of Perception* (New York: Routledge, 1999 [1962]); Erving Goffman, *Behaviour in Public* (London: Allen Lane, 1963); *Interaction Ritual: Essays on Face-to-Face Behaviour* (Garden City, N.Y.: Doubleday, 1968); and *Stigma: Notes on the Management of Spoiled Identity* (Harmondsworth: Penguin, 1968 [1963]).

20. Simon J. Williams and Gillian A. Bendelow, *The Lived Body*, 3.

21. Simon J. Williams and Gillian A. Bendelow, *The Lived Body*, 3, emphasis in original.

22. From this notion that controllability of the body exists arises the idea that persons with chronic pain are "uncontrollable."

23. We discuss this in more detail below.

24. Examples include Mary Ann O'Farrell and Lynne Vallone, eds., *Virtual Gender: Fantasies of Subjectivity and Embodiment* (Ann Arbor: University of Michigan Press, 1999); Malin Pereira, *Embodying Beauty: Twentieth-century American Women Writers' Aesthetics* (New York: Garland, 2000); Debra Walker King, ed., *Body Politics and the Fictional Double* (Bloomington: Indiana University Press, 2000); Jocalyn Lawler, *Behind the Screens: Nursing, Somology, and the Problem of the Body*, North American edition (Redwood City, Calif.: Benjamin/Cummings, 1993); Patricia Benner, ed., *Interpretive Phenomenology: Embodiment, Caring, and Ethics in Health and Illness* (Thousand Oaks, Calif.: Sage, 1994); Patricia Benner, "The Roles of Embodiment, Emotion, and Lifeworld for Rationality and Agency in Nursing Practice," *Nursing Philosophy* 1, no. 1 (2000): 5–19; James B. Nelson, *Body Theology* (Louisville: Westminster/John Knox Press, 1988); Naomi R. Goldenberg, *Resurrecting the Body: Feminism, Religion, and Psychoanalysis* (New York: Crossroad, 1993); and Lisa Isherwood, *The Good News of the Body: Sexual Theology and Feminism* (Sheffield, U.K.: Sheffield University Press, 2000).

25. There are other works that have influenced our understanding of self, subjectivity, and identity, but in different ways. Anne Ferguson, *Blood at the Root: Motherhood, Sexuality, and Male Dominance* (London: Pandora, 1989); Mary O'Brien, *The Politics of Reproduction* (London: Routledge and Kegan Paul, 1981); and Lise Vogel, *Marxism and the Oppression of Women: Toward a Unitary Theory* (New Brunswick, N.J.: Rutgers University Press, 1983) have been significant in shaping how we see the materiality of the economy play out in women's lives. More recently, Teresa Ebert, *Ludic Feminism and After: Postmodernism, Desire, and Labor in Late Capitalism* (Ann Arbor: University of Michigan Press, 1996) has reminded us that discourse and materiality are not the same, and not everything can be reduced to text. We

bleed, we hurt, we die. The context within which we bleed, hurt, and die is only as important as the material conditions giving rise to these acts and states of beings. Feminist materialism still holds its own as a strong influence in feminist theory, especially in relation to explaining women's labor, both paid and unpaid. See, for example, Rosemary Pringle, *Secretaries Talk: Sexuality, Power, and Work* (London: Verso, 1989); Rosemary Crompton and Kay Sanderson, *Gendered Jobs and Social Change* (London: Unwin Hyman, 1990); Cynthia Cockburn, *Brothers: Male Dominance and Technological Change* (London: Pluto Press, 1990); and Sylvia Walby, *Gender Transformations* (New York: Routledge, 1996). Other works outside labor include examples in Rosemary Hennessy and Chrys Ingraham, eds., *Materialist Feminism: A Reader in Class, Difference, and Women's Lives* (New York: Routledge, 1995); Kathryn Russel, "A Value-Theoretic Approach to Childbirth and Reproductive Engineering," 328–44; Meera Nanda, " 'History Is What Hurts': A Materialist Feminist Perspective on the Green Revolution and Its Ecofeminist Critics," 364–94; and Cynthia R. Comacchio, "Motherhood in Crisis: Women, Medicine, and State in Canada 1900–1940," 306–27.

One problematic we have found with this approach in the literature is that there is little room outside the construct of class and a meso-scale to develop an analysis that can account for an individual woman's experiences of illness. What matters for us here is the entwinement of the material—not only the economic or material conditions of bodily existence but also the biological make-up, anatomical structure, and the physiological processes that also constitute the body.

26. Elizabeth Grosz, "Psychoanalysis and the Body," in *Feminist Theory and the Body: A Reader*, ed. Janet Price and Margrit Shildrick (New York: Routledge, 1998), 270, emphasis in original.

27. This is the argument Iris Marion Young lays out in "The Scaling of Bodies and the Politics of Identity," in *Justice and the Politics of Difference* (Princeton: Princeton University Press, 1990), 122–55.

28. Object relations theory is an obvious example.

29. This is true of Elizabeth Grosz, Iris Marion Young, and Judith Butler. This is the source of extreme frustration for materialist feminists who have drawn intellectual directions from both Western Marxism and northern feminism.

30. Judith Butler, *Gender Trouble*, and Jana Sawicki, *Disciplining Foucault: Feminism, Power, and the Body* (New York: Routledge, 1991).

31. Michel Foucault, *Discipline and Punish: The Birth of the Prison* (New York: Vintage, 1979), *The History of Sexuality, An Introduction, Volume 1* (New York: Vintage, 1978), and *The History of Sexuality, Volume 3: The Care of the Self* (New York: Vintage, 1988).

32. Judith Butler, *Gender Trouble*, 13.

33. Judith Butler, *Gender Trouble*, 24.

34. Judith Butler, *Gender Trouble*, 25.

35. Judith Butler, *Gender Trouble*, 148.

36. Jana Sawicki, *Disciplining Foucault*, 1.

37. Jana Sawicki, *Disciplining Foucault*, 55 and 56.

38. Jana Sawicki, *Disciplining Foucault*, 100.

39. Jana Sawicki, *Disciplining Foucault*, 95 and 103–5.

40. Part of our unsteadiness in "fixing" our objections stems from the way in which works like these have been criticized for being too abstract and apolitical. However, Judith Butler makes her arguments more specific in *Bodies That Matter: On the Discursive Limits of "Sex"* (New York: Routledge, 1993) and discusses politics in *Excitable Speech: A Politics of the Performative* (New York: Routledge, 1997).

41. Julia Cream, "Women on Trial: A Private Pillory?" in *Mapping the Subject: Geographies of Cultural Transformation*, ed. Steve Pile and Nigel Thrift (New York: Routledge, 1995), 158–69, argues that performing womanhood with the "pill" has been experienced variously by groups of women depending on their social locations—family planning, sexual liberation, or exploited economically for drug production and physically through drug testing.

42. Elspeth Probyn, *Sexing the Self*.

43. Including, for example, Michel Foucault, *The History of Sexuality, Volume 1*; *The History of Sexuality, Volume 2: The Use of Pleasure* (New York: Vintage, 1990); *The Care of the Self*; and *Herculine Barbin: Being the Recently Discovered Memoirs of a Nineteenth-century French Hermaphrodite* (Brighton: Harvester Press, 1980).

44. Elspeth Probyn, *Sexing the Self*, 55.

45. Elspeth Probyn, *Sexing the Self*, 80.

46. Elspeth Probyn, *Sexing the Self*, 128.

47. Elspeth Probyn draws on Foucault's notion of attitude in "What Is Enlightenment?" in *The Foucault Reader*, ed. Paul Rabinow (New York: Pantheon, 1984), 32–50.

48. Elspeth Probyn, *Sexing the Self*, 138.

49. Elspeth Probyn, *Sexing the Self*, 172.

50. Michel Foucault, *Archaeology of Knowledge* (New York: Routledge, 1972), 107, and *History of Sexuality, Volume 1*, 100–2.

51. The collection of works edited by Sarah Nettleton and Jonathan Watson, *The Body in Everyday Life* (New York: Routledge, 1997) contains several good examples of how discourses about the body define and give meaning to the body, including especially Alexandra Howson, "Embodied Obligation: The Female Body and Health Surveillance," 218–40; and Eileen Fairhurst, " 'Growing Old Gracefully' as Opposed to 'Mutton Dressed as Lamb': The Social Construction of Recognising Older Women," 258–75. So, too, does the collection edited by Elizabeth Grosz and Elspeth Probyn, *Sexy Bodies: The Strange Carnalities of Feminism* (New York: Routledge, 1995), especially Melissa Jane Hardie, " 'I Embrace the Difference': Elizabeth Taylor and the Closet," 155–71.

52. In a classic series of essays, Emily Martin, *The Woman in the Body: A Cultural Analysis of Reproduction*, 2nd ed. (Boston: Beacon Press, 1992) shows how meanings ascribed to reproductive bodily processes shape women and their bodies and have material consequences.

53. In both the introductions to each section as well as the pieces themselves, Cherríe Moraga and Gloria Anzaldúa, eds., *This Bridge Called My Back: Writings by Radical Women of Color* (New York: Kitchen Table Press, 1986) make this point over and over again quite dramatically.

54. For example, Iris Marion Young, *Throwing Like a Girl and Other Essays* (Bloomington: Indiana University Press, 1990); Gayatri Chakravorty Spivak, "Can

the Subaltern Speak?" in *Colonial Discourses and Post-Colonial Theory: A Reader*, ed. Patrick Williams and Laura Chrisman (Hertfordshire, U.K.: Harvester Wheatsheaf, 1994), 66–112; and Chantal Mouffe, "Feminism, Citizenship, and Radical Democratic Politics," in *Feminists Theorize the Political*, ed. Judith Butler and Joan W. Scott (New York: Routledge, 1992), 369–84 among others.

55. For applications, see for example, Anna Yeatman, "A Feminist Theory of Social Differentiation," in *Feminism/Postmodernism*, ed. Linda J. Nicholson (New York: Routledge, 1990), 281–99; Karen J. Swift and Michael Birmingham, "Location, Location, Location: Restructuring and the Everyday Lives of 'Welfare Moms,'" in *Restructuring Caring Labour: Discourse, State Practice, and Everyday Life*, ed. Sheila M. Neysmith (Toronto: Oxford University Press, 2000), 93–115; and Judith Butler, *Gender Trouble*.

56. Although this is not always the case. For example, see studies of national identity, Liisa Malkki, "Refugees and Exile: From 'Refugee Studies' to the National Order of Things," *Annual Review of Anthropology* 24 (1995): 495–524; Joanne P. Sharp, "Gendering Nationhood: A Feminist Engagement with National Identity," in *Body/Space: Destabilizing Geographies of Gender and Sexuality*, ed. Nancy Duncan (New York: Routledge, 1996), 97–108; and Nira Yuval-Davis, *Gender and Nation* (London: Sage, 1997).

57. Mouffe's argument as we have laid it out here can be found in Chantal Mouffe, "Feminism, Citizenship, and Radical Democratic Politics," 370–73 and in "Post-Marxism, Democracy and Identity," *Environment and Planning D: Society and Space* 13 (1995): 259–65.

58. We drew this out of Clare Hemmings, "Locating Bisexual Identities: Discourses of Bisexuality and Contemporary Feminist Theory," in *Mapping Desires*, ed. David Bell and Gill Valentine (New York: Routledge, 1995), 41–55, even though she does not explicitly make this argument.

59. Although embryonic, we think that this theoretical direction may be more useful than the existing alternatives for theorizing bisexuality in queer and feminist theory, as for example, Elizabeth Wilson, "Is Transgression Transgressive?" in *Activating Theory: Lesbian, Gay, Bisexual Politics*, ed. Joseph Bristow and Angelia R. Wilson (London: Lawrence and Wishart, 1993), 107–17. This type of theorization—where one has to be either heterosexual or homosexual—appears fairly often in the psychoanalytic theory literature, particularly around therapy. For example, three authors in *Disorienting Sexuality: Psychoanalytic Reappraisals of Sexual Identities*, ed. Thomas Domenici and Ronnie C. Lesser (New York: Routledge, 1995) mention bisexuality in passing. Ronnie C. Lesser, in "Objectivity as Masquerade," 83–96, discusses a debate wherein a bisexual man, considered ambivalent about his sexuality, was treated successfully because after therapy he was heterosexual. Although not the focus of the argument, Lesser does not take up the issue of there being no space for bisexuality in his arguments about the myth of objectivity in both theory and therapy. A similar move takes place by Robert May, in "Re-Reading Freud on Homosexuality," 153–65. He comments that Freud jettisoned bisexuality in favor of a "normative notion of health" (154) but does not follow up with more detailed analysis. This is ironic given that the central thesis of his piece is that Freud set up psychoanalysis as a process of "self-dissolving categories," "posing and merging

opposites," "the repeated creation of collapse of meaning," and "the endless undoing of certainty" (162). Finally, Mark J. Blecher, in "The Shaping of Psychoanalytic
Theory and Practice," 265–88, reads Lesser's comments and proposes that bisexuality is in opposition to monosexuality, a category not pathologized in psychoanalysis.
This is more of a step toward "disorienting sexuality," especially if it means more
than just legitimating homosexuality, whereby opening up analysis of expressions of
sexuality means challenging the hegemony of binary discourse. For more complex
theorizations of bisexuality, see John Money, *Gay, Straight and In-Between: Sexology
of Erotic Orientation* (New York: Oxford University Press, 1988); Marjorie J.
Garber, *Bisexuality and the Eroticism of Everyday Life* (New York: Routledge, 2000)
[originally published as *Vice Versa: Bisexuality and the Eroticism of Everyday Life*
(New York: Simon and Schuster, 1995)]; and Paula C. Rodríguez Rust, "Bisexuality: A Contemporary Paradox for Women," *Journal of Social Issues* 56, no. 2 (2000):
205–21. Also, contributions in Merl Storr, ed., *Bisexuality: A Critical Reader* (New
York: Routledge, 2000) explore bisexuality as it is rather than what it is not.

60. Iris Marion Young, "The Ideal of Community and the Politics of Difference," in *Feminism/Postmodernism*, 319.

61. Pamela Moss, " 'Not Quite Abled, Not Quite Disabled: Experiences of
Being 'In Between' ME and the Academy," *Disability Studies Quarterly* 20 (2000):
287–93 extends this argument in analyzing her own experiences within the
academy.

NOTES FOR CHAPTER 3

1. At the same time, we are challenged to maintain our interests in space empirically and theoretically in our scholarship and teaching, because, at the time of writing this book, we are both located outside social science disciplines in professional
faculties associated with health and social services.

2. Works on the body that are based on humanist values and have dominated
the shaping of how illness is approached analytically in the social sciences include,
for example, Arthur Frank, *At the Will of the Body* (Boston: Houghton Mifflin,
1991) and *The Wounded Storyteller: Body, Illness, and Ethics* (Chicago: University of
Chicago Press, 1995); Arthur Kleinman, *The Illness Narratives: Suffering, Healing
and the Human Condition* (New York: Basic, 1988); and Kathy Charmaz, *Good
Days, Bad Days* (New Brunswick, N.J.: Rutgers University Press, 1991). Even in
critiques, as for example Douglas Ezzy, "Illness Narratives: Time, Hope and HIV,"
Social Science and Medicine 50 (2000): 605–17, humanist values are still prominent.

3. For examples, see Michael Bury, "Chronic Illness as Biographical Disrup-
tion," *Sociology of Health and Illness* 4, no. 2 (1982): 167–82; Sharon Kaufman,
"Illness, Biography, and the Interpretation of Self Following a Stroke," *Journal of
Aging Studies* 2, no. 3 (1988): 217–27; and Ian Robinson, "Personal Narratives,
Social Careers, and Medical Courses: Analysing Life Trajectories in Autobiographies
of People with Multiple Sclerosis," *Social Science and Medicine* 30 (1990): 1173–86.

4. As an example, see Douglas Ezzy, "Lived Experience and Interpretation in

Narrative Theory: Experience of Living with HIV/AIDS," *Qualitative Sociology* 21 (1998): 169–80.

5. Joan W. Scott, " 'Experience,' " in *Feminists Theorize the Political*, ed. Judith Butler and Joan W. Scott (New York: Routledge, 1992), 37, emphasis in original. (Originally appeared as "Experience," *Critical Inquiry*, (summer, 1991): 773–97.)

6. It is imperative to note that in conceiving experience as a contestable interpretation we are not justifying any concrete actions of interpretation whether they be physicians' claims that many of the experiences of women with chronic illness are psychosomatic or some other ostensibly malevolent act that denies women's experiences. Indeed, by conceiving experience as an interpretation, we can explain how competing interpretations of illness—that of the biomedical physician and that of the woman experiencing chronic illness—emerge to shape women's experiences of being chronically ill.

7. We extend these thoughts in the following chapter wherein we outline in more detail our conceptual framework. For now, we focus on the refusing of the discursive as either separate from or the same as the material.

8. For example, Heidi Nast, "Opening Remarks on 'Women in the Field,' " *Professional Geographer* 46 (1994): 54–66; Cindi Katz, "Playing the Field: Questions of Fieldwork in Geography," *Professional Geographer* 46 (1994): 67–72.

9. This state of "in betweenness" is developed analytically in terms of chronic illness by Pamela Moss, "Not Quite Abled, Not Quite Disabled: Experiences of Being 'In Between' ME and the Academy," *Disability Studies Quarterly* 20 (2000): 287–93 and in terms of difference by Heidi Nast, "Opening Remarks."

10. Literature on women's health varies widely, ranging from disease incidence studies to creating an ethic of care. Issues rooted in the struggle of the control of women's bodies have provided the foundation for the early emergence of feminist studies of women's health, as for example, birth control, reproductive rights, and abortion. The landmark book, *Our Bodies, Ourselves: A Book By and For Women*, by the Boston Women's Health Book Collective (New York: Simon and Schuster, 1973) initiated an era of women's demands to have a say in the care of their bodies. (The book was updated and reissued in 1992 by the same publisher.) By the mid- to late-1990s, throughout Canada and the United States, there was an upsurge of interest in designating women's health concerns as a priority in research and health care delivery. Government funding in collaboration with universities and research institutes established several Centers of Excellence for Women's Health across the continent in cities such as Ann Arbor, Boston, Chicago, Columbus, Halifax, Indianapolis, Los Angeles, Montreal, Philadelphia, San Francisco, Toronto, Vancouver, and Winnipeg. Although these centers support gender-sensitive research and care provision, there is no guarantee that there is a feminist analysis. In fact, most of the centers are closely linked to medical training and research institutes.

Much work on women's health and illness in the social sciences has focused on understanding the social construction of women and their social needs (see Simon J. Williams and Gillian A. Bendelow, "Bodily Control: Body Techniques, Intercorporeality and the Embodiment of Social Action," 49–66; and "Pain and the Dys-Appearing Body," in *The Lived Body: Sociological Themes, Embodied Issue*, 155–70, New York: Routledge, 1998). But it is not only the social construction of femaleness and womanhood that is at issue; it is also the woman in the body, meaning the materiality of the woman's existence (see Emily Martin, *The Woman in the Body: A Cultural Analysis of Reproduction*, 2nd ed., Boston: Beacon Press, 1992). In geography, interest in women's health expanded with Michael Dorn and Glenda Laws' plea for a more *embodied* geography in "Social Theory, Body Politics, and Medical Geography: Extending Kearns's Invitation," *Professional Geographer* 46, no. 1 (1994): 106–10. A collection of articles in *Geoforum* 26, no. 3 (1995): 239–323, showed a wide range of interests, social policy, quality and access to medical care, and cultural difference; see Carolyn Gallaher, "Social Policy and the Construction of Need: A Critical Examination of the Geography of Needs Assessments for Low-income Women's Health," 287–96; Mary M. Flad, "Tracing an Irish Widow's Journey: Immigration and Medical Care in the Mid-nineteenth Century," 261–72; Isabel Dyck, "Putting Chronic Illness 'In Place': Women Immigrants' Accounts of Their Health Care," 247–60; and Sara McLafferty and Barbara Tempalski, "Restructuring and Women's Reproductive Health: Implications for Low Birthweight in New York City," 309–323. More recently, interesting works have been collected in volumes edited by Ruth Butler and Hester Parr, eds. *Mind and Body Spaces: Geographies of Illness, Impairment and Disability* (New York: Routledge, 1999) and by Isabel Dyck, Nancy Davis Lewis, and Sara McLafferty, eds., *Geographies of Women's Health* (New York: Routledge, 2001).

11. Hester Parr, "Bodies and Psychiatric Medicine: Interpreting Different Geographies of Mental Health," in *Mind and Body Spaces*, 189.

12. Jennifer Terry, "Anxious Slippages between 'Us' and 'Them': A Brief History of the Scientific Search for Homosexual Bodies," in *Deviant Bodies*, ed. Jennifer Terry and Jacqueline Urla (Bloomington: Indiana University press, 1995), 129–69.

13. Jennifer Terry, "Anxious Slippages between 'Us' and 'Them,' " 152.

14. Cited in Jennifer Terry, "Anxious Slippages between 'Us' and 'Them,' " 155 and 157.

15. Jennifer Terry, "Anxious Slippages between 'Us' and 'Them,' " 161.

16. Jennifer Terry, "Anxious Slippages between 'Us' and 'Them,' " 158 and 161.

17. Diane Price Herndl, *Invalid Women: Figuring Feminine Illness in American Fiction and Culture, 1840–1940* (Chapel Hill: University of North Carolina Press, 1993).

18. Diane Price Herndl, *Invalid Women*, 220.

19. Susan E. Abbey and Paul E. Garfinkel, "Neurasthenia and Chronic Fatigue Syndrome: The Role of Culture in the Making of a Diagnosis," *American Journal of Psychiatry* 148, no. 12 (December 1991): 1638–46.

20. Susan E. Abbey and Paul E. Garfinkel, "Neurasthenia and Chronic Fatigue Syndrome," 1644.

21. We do not take up a critique of this argument.

22. This is a theme taken up by Elaine Showalter, *Hystories: Hysterical Epidemics and Modern Media* (New York: Columbia University Press, 1997) wherein she compares the anxiety with Chronic Fatigue Syndrome with other end of the millennium bodily phenomena. We discuss this in detail in chapter 2, note 8.

23. Vivienne Anderson, "A Will of Its Own: Experiencing the Body in Severe Chronic Illness," in *Women's Bodies/Women's Lives: Health, Well-Being and Body*

Image, ed. Baukje Miedema, Janet M. Stoppard, and Vivienne Anderson (Toronto: Sumach Press, 2000), 29–41. Scleroderma is a systemic autoimmune disease that destroys soft tissue.

24. But only to a point. The ongoing fluctuations with chronic illness are difficult to accept for family and friends, and often harder to accommodate. We discuss this further in chapters 8 and 9.

25. Heidi Nast and Steve Pile, "Introduction: MakingPlaceBodies," in *Places through the Body*, ed. Heidi J. Nast and Steve Pile (New York: Routledge, 1998), 6.

26. Armando R. Favazza, *Bodies under Siege: Self-Mutilation and Body Modification in Culture and Psychiatry* (Baltimore: Johns Hopkins University Press, 1996).

27. Fakir Musafar, "Body Play: State of Grace or Sickness?" in *Bodies under Siege*, 325–34.

28. As they would be in "unity."

29. Kathy Davis, *Reshaping the Female Body: The Dilemma of Cosmetic Surgery* (New York: Routledge, 1995).

30. Susan Bordo, *Unbearable Weight: Feminism, Western Culture, and the Body* (Berkeley: University of California Press, 1993), 67.

31. Susan Bordo, *Unbearable Weight*, 68.

32. Abigail Bray and Claire Colebrook, "The Haunted Flesh: Corporeal Feminism and the Politics of (Dis)Embodiment," *Signs* 24, no. 1 (1998): 35–67.

33. Elizabeth Grosz makes this argument in *Volatile Bodies: Toward a Corporeal Feminism* (Bloomington: Indiana University Press, 1994), 40.

34. As laid out by Gilles Deleuze, *Difference and Repetition*, trans. Paul Patton (New York: Columbia University, 1994).

35. Abigail Bray and Claire Colebrook, "The Haunted Flesh," 62.

36. Abigail Bray and Claire Colebrook, "The Haunted Flesh," 63.

37. Kelvyn Jones and Graham Moon, "Medical Geography: Taking Space Seriously," *Progress in Human Geography* 17 (1993): 515–24.

38. John Eyles, "From Disease Ecology and Spatial Analysis to . . . ? The Challenges of Medical Geography in Canada," *Health and Canadian Society* 1, no. 1 (1993): 113–45

39. Robin A. Kearns and Alun E. Joseph, "Space in Its Place: Developing the Link in Medical Geography," *Social Science and Medicine* 37, no. 6 (1993): 711–17.

40. Robin A. Kearns and Alun E. Joseph, "Space in Its Place," 716.

41. Researchers and analysts involved in medical geography became dissatisfied with the close and obvious connection with medicine. In an attempt to distance themselves, at least ideologically, from biomedical models of health and illness and from simplistic conceptualizations associated with the sub-discipline, medical geographers increasingly identify themselves as working in the field of geography of health and health care, or simply health geographers. This movement no doubt was influenced by the increased engagement by some health geographers with social theory and other critical approaches. The founding of the journal *Health and Place*, with its inaugural issue January 1995, is evidence of this shift.

42. For examples, see Doreen Massey, *Spatial Divisions of Labour* (London: Macmillan, 1984) and Michael Storper and Richard Walker, *The Capitalist Imperative* (London: Blackwell, 1989).

43. David Wilson and Pamela Moss, "Spatiality Studies in Urban Geography," in *Research in Urban Sociology, vol. 4*, ed. Ray Hutchinson (Greenwich, Conn.: JAI Press, 1997), 3.

44. Edward W. Soja, "The Socio-Spatial Dialectic," *Annals of the Association of American Geographers* 70 (1980): 207–25.

45. Henri Lefebvre, *The Everyday Life of the Modern World* (Middlesex: Penguin, 1968) [English translation 1972] and *The Urban Revolution* (Paris: Gallimard, 1970).

46. Edward W. Soja, "The Trialectics of Spatiality," in *Thirdspace: Journeys to Los Angeles and Other Real-And-Imagined Places* (London: Blackwell, 1996), 53–82.

47. Steve Pile, "Human Agency and Human Geography Revisited: A Critique of 'New Models' of the Self," *Transactions of the Institute of British Geographers* 18 (1993): 122–39. See also Michael Keith and Steve Pile, eds., *Place and the Politics of Identity* (New York: Routledge, 1993); Steve Pile and Nigel Thrift, introduction to *Mapping the Subject: Geographies of Cultural Transformation*, ed. Steve Pile and Nigel Thrift (New York: Routledge, 1995), 1–12; and Steve Pile, *The Body and the City: Psychoanalysis, Space, and Subjectivity* (New York: Routledge, 1996).

48. Doreen Massey, "A Global Sense of Place."

49. Elizabeth Grosz, "Bodies-Cities," in *Space, Time, and Perversion* (New York: Routledge, 1995), 103–10.

50. Elizabeth Grosz, "Bodies-Cities," 108.

51. Heidi J. Nast, "The Body as 'Place': Reflexivity and Fieldwork in Kano, Nigeria," in *Places through the Body*, 93–116. Her main point here is to conceive the body-as-place, collapse the two into one another, a theoretical position that contradicts our claim of simultaneity in lieu of unity.

52. *Bayi* is Hausa for slave.

53. Critical studies across the academy abound with spatial phrases to describe a process, as for example, "mapping the postmodern," "creating space for voice," or "locating identity politics." See, for example, Andreas Huyssen, "Mapping the Postmodern," in *Feminism/Postmodernism*, ed. Linda J. Nicholson (New York: Routledge, 1990), 234–77; Elspeth Probyn, "Travels in the Postmodern: Making Sense of the Local," in *Feminism/Postmodernism*, 176–89; and Liz Bondi, "Locating Identity Politics," *Place and the Politics of Identity*, 84–101. Spatial metaphors also comprise theoretical constructs, as for example, paradoxical space (Gillian Rose, *Feminism and Geography: The Limits of Geographical Knowledge*, Minneapolis: University of Minnesota Press, 1993), territoriality and deterritorialization (Gilles Deleuze and Félix Guattari, *A Thousand Plateaus*, Minneapolis: University of Minnesota Press, 1987), and *habitus* (Pierre Bourdieu, *Outline of a Theory of Practice*, Cambridge: Cambridge University Press, 1977). For a discussion of the uses of spatial metaphors, see Trevor Barnes and James Duncan, eds., *Writing Worlds: Discourse, Text, and Metaphor in the Representation of Landscape* (New York: Routledge, 1992). For non-feminist examples of spatializing epistemologies, see Paul Routledge, "The Third Space as Critical Engagement," *Antipode* 28 (1996): 399–419; and Andrew Jones, "(Re)producing Gender Relations," *Geoforum* 29 (1999): 451–74.

54. Liz Bondi, "Locating Identity Politics."

55. Liz Bondi, "Locating Identity Politics," 98; Diana Fuss, *Essentially Speaking* (New York: Routledge, 1989).

56. Liz Bondi, "Locating Identity Politics," 98.

57. Colin Gordon, "Afterward," in *Power/Knowledge: Selected Interviews and Other Writings, 1972–1977* (New York: Pantheon, 1980), 233.

58. See Jana Sawicki, *Disciplining Foucault: Feminism, Power, and the Body* (New York: Routledge, 1991).

59. Michel Foucault, "Questions on Geography," in *Power/Knowledge*, 77.

60. Michel Foucault, "Questions on Geography," 77.

61. Notions of partiality permeate literature in feminist epistemology, especially in geography. Most of this work derives from Donna Haraway, "Situated Knowledges: The Science Question in Feminism and the Privilege of Partial Perspective," *Feminist Studies* 14, no. 3 (1998): 575–99. She argues that "politics and epistemologies of location, positioning, and situating, where partiality and not universality is the condition of being heard to make rational knowledge claims. These are claims on people's lives. I am arguing for the view from a body, always a complex, contradictory, structuring, and structured body, versus the view from above, from nowhere, from simplicity. Only the god trick is forbidden. Here is a criterion for deciding the science question in militarism, that dream science/technology of perfect language, perfect communication, final order" (589).

NOTES FOR CHAPTER 4

1. By deployment, we do not mean that power is something to "hold" and then to be "dispensed" in order to control or oppress other people. Rather, power is something exercised and emerges through interaction generated by "bodies in context." As we discuss later in this chapter, these deployments of power have normalizing and naturalizing tendencies that discipline and regulate bodies.

2. We discuss "corporeal space" in the context of the diagnosis process in Pamela Moss and Isabel Dyck, "Body, Corporeal Space, and Legitimating Chronic Illness: Women Diagnosed with M.E.," *Antipode* 31 (1999): 372–97.

3. See discussion of spatiality in chapter 3.

4. Pamela Moss and Isabel Dyck, "Material Bodies Precariously Positioned: Women Embodying Chronic Illness in the Workplace," in *Geographies of Women's Health*, ed. Isabel Dyck, Nancy Davis Lewis, and Sara McLafferty (New York: Routledge, 2001), 232.

5. We have drawn this formulation of inscription from a number of sources including Gelya Frank, "On Embodiment: A Case of Congenital Limb Deficiency in American Culture," in *Women with Disabilities: Essays in Psychology, Culture, and Politics*, ed. Michelle Fine and Adrienne Asch (Philadelphia: Temple University Press, 1988), 41–71; Judith Butler, "Foucault and the Paradox of Bodily Inscriptions," *The Journal of Philosophy* 86, no. 11 (1989): 601–7; and Elizabeth Grosz, "Inscriptions and Body-maps: Representations and the Corporeal," in *Feminine, Masculine, and Representation*, ed. Terry Threadgold and Anne Cranny-Francis (Sydney, Aus.: Allen and Unwin, 1990), 62–74; and her extension of this work in "Body Images: Neurophysiology and Corporeal Mappings" and "The Body as Inscriptive Surface," in *Volatile Bodies: Toward a Corporeal Feminism* (Bloomington: Indiana

University Press, 1994), 62–85 and 138–59. Although not specifically about inscription, Ursula Sharma's theoretical work around dualistic thinking in "Bringing the Body Back into the (Social) Action: Techniques of the Body and the (Cultural) Imagination," *Social Anthropology* 4, no. 3 (1996): 251–63, was helpful in sorting through the imagined aspects of what inscriptions might be.

6. Linda McDowell, in *Gender, Identity, and Space: Understanding Feminist Geographies* (Cambridge: Polity Press, 1999), organized her book-length review of feminist geography according to scale, with the body being the smallest and nation, the largest. There are more sophisticated conceptualizations of scale in the geography literature, as for example, the constructionist perspective of scale outlined by David Delaney and Helga Leitner in "The Political Construction of Scale," *Political Geography* 16, no. 2 (1997): 93–97.

7. The links to the formulation of the project are discussed further in chapter 5.

8. Joan W. Scott, " 'Experience,' " in *Feminists Theorize the Political*, ed. Judith Butler and Joan W. Scott (New York: Routledge, 1992).

9. Theresa Ebert, *Ludic Feminism and After: Postmodernism, Desire, and Labor in Late Capitalism* (Ann Arbor: University of Michigan Press, 1996).

10. Ebert, *Ludic Feminism*, 13.

11. Ebert, *Ludic Feminism*, 13.

12. Ebert, *Ludic Feminism*, 13.

13. See especially Pamela Moss, "Autobiographical Notes on Chronic Illness," in *Mind and Body Spaces: Geographies of Disability, Illness, and Impairment*, ed. Ruth Butler and Hester Parr (New York: Routledge, 1999), 155–66, and "Not Quite Abled and Not Quite Disabled: Experiences of Being 'In Between' ME and the Academy," *Disability Studies Quarterly* 20, no. 3 (2000): 787–93. Susan Wendell uses autobiographical writing to draw out issues concerning theorizing disability from her experiences of being ill with chronic illness in *The Rejected Body: Feminist Philosophical Reflections on Disability* (New York: Routledge, 1996).

14. See Sue Wise, "Sexing Elvis," *Women's Studies International Forum* 7, no. 1 (1984): 13–17. An effective example in geography is Liz Bondi's work in her ongoing study of the interconnections between psychotherapeutic practices and human geography, as represented in "Stages on Journeys: Some Remarks about Human Geography and Psychotherapeutic Practice," *Professional Geographer* 51 (1999): 11–24. She weaves autobiographical accounts of her experiences of working as a feminist academic with theories of a de-centered, fragmented self and as an unhappy person engaged in psychotherapy rooted in humanist values. She uses this work to demonstrate the need for a space for setting up a dialogue among competing frameworks and difference in meanings.

15. For example, see Arthur Frank, *The Wounded Storyteller: Body, Illness, and Ethics* (Chicago: University of Chicago Press, 1995) and Thomas J. Csordas, ed., *Embodiment and Experience: The Existential Ground of Culture and Self* (New York: Cambridge University Press, 1994). Other collections draw on a wide range of philosophical underpinnings, including spirituality, as for example, Kat Duff, *The Alchemy of Illness* (London: Virago, 1994) and the special issue on serious illness in *Holistic Nursing Practice* 12, no. 1.

16. Margrit Shildrick and Janet Price, "Breaking the Boundaries of the Broken Body," *Body and Society* 2, no. 4 (1996): 93–113.

17. Shildrick and Price, "Breaking the Boundaries of the Broken Body," 113.

18. Some examples of these works include Paul A. Komesaroff, ed., *Troubled Bodies: Critical Perspectives on Postmodernism, Medical Ethics, and the Body* (Durham, N.C.: Duke University Press, 1995); Gail Weiss, *Body Images: Embodiment as Intercorporeality* (New York: Routledge, 1999); and Angela Keane and Avril Horner, *Body Matters: Feminism, Textuality, Corporeality* (Manchester, U.K.: Manchester University Press, 2000).

19. David Harvey, "The Body as an Accumulation Strategy," *Environment & Planning D: Society & Space* 16 (1998): 401–21; and Felicity J. Callard, "The Body in Theory," *Environment & Planning D: Society & Space* 16 (1998): 387–400. These are not the only works that seek to embody political economy. See also Deborah Leslie and David Butz, " 'GM Suicide': Flexibility, Space, and the Injured Body," *Economic Geography* 74 (1998): 360–78; Patricia L. Price, "Bodies, Faith, and Inner Landscapes: Rethinking Change from the Very Local," *Latin American Perspectives* 26, no. 3 (1999): 37–59; and Brooke Grundfest Schoepf, "Inscribing the Body Politic: Women and AIDS in Africa," in *Pragmatic Women and Body Politics*, ed. Margaret Lock and Patricia A. Kaufert, 98–125 (Cambridge: Cambridge University Press, 1998).

20. Seyla Benhabib, "The Generalized and the Concrete Other: The Kohlberg-Gilligan Controversy and Moral Theory," in *Situating the Self: Gender, Community and Postmodernism in Contemporary Ethics* (New York: Routledge, 1992), 152, emphasis in the original.

21. Elizabeth Grosz, *Volatile Bodies: Toward a Corporeal Feminism* (Bloomington: Indiana University Press, 1994), 209.

22. Most notably Judith Butler, *Gender Trouble: Feminism and the Subversion of Identity* (New York: Routledge, 1990) and *Bodies That Matter: On the Discursive Limits of "Sex"* (New York: Routledge, 1993).

23. Abigail Bray and Claire Colebrook, "The Haunted Flesh: Corporeal Feminism and the Politics of (Dis)Embodiment," *Signs* 24, no. 1 (1998): 35–67.

24. Abigail Bray and Claire Colebrook, "The Haunted Flesh," 36.

25. Abigail Bray and Claire Colebrook, "The Haunted Flesh," 37.

26. Thus far we have been focusing on a critique of the pre-discursive body. In congruence with our arguments around challenging the dichotomy of discourse and materiality, we also want to make a point of refusing a pre-mattered body—querying the notion that there is a non-material body prior to a fleshed one.

27. Alexandra Howson, "Embodied Obligation: The Female Body and Health Surveillance," in *The Body in Everyday Life*, ed. Sarah Nettleton and Jonathan Watson, 218–40 (New York: Routledge, 1999).

28. Alexandra Howson, "Embodied Obligation," 226.

29. Alexandra Howson, "Embodied Obligation," 219, our emphasis for definition. See Bryan S. Turner, *Medical Power and Social Knowledge* (London: Sage, 1995 [1987]).

30. Michel Foucault, *Discipline and Punish: The Birth of a Prison* (New York: Vintage, 1979) and *The Birth of the Clinic: An Archaeology of Medical Perception* (New York: Vintage, 1973).

31. Michel Foucault, *Discipline and Punish*, 138.

32. Michel Foucault, *Discipline and Punish*, 308
33. Michel Foucault, *Discipline and Punish*, 306.
34. Michel Foucault, *Discipline and Punish*, 306.
35. Michel Foucault, *The Birth of the Clinic*, 196.
36. Michel Foucault, *The Birth of the Clinic*, 199.
37. It is difficult at this point not to mention that many Marxists have severe reservations about the ability for Foucault's theory to deal adequately with the differentiation of the constitutive subject. These concerns are articulated concisely in Eleanor MacDonald, "The Trouble with Subjects: Feminism, Marxism and the Questions of Poststructuralism," *Studies in Political Economy* 35 (1991): 43–71 and David Michael Levin, "The Body Politic: The Embodiment of Praxis in Foucault and Habermas," *Praxis International* 9, nos. 1 and 2 (July 1989): 112–32.

What concerns us more is the difficulties feminists have with Foucault's theories. As we discussed in chapters 2 and 3, Jana Sawicki, in *Disciplining Foucault: Feminism, Power, and the Body* (New York: Routledge, 1991), challenges Foucault's interpretation of resistance. In a collection of feminist writings, Caroline Ramazanoglu, *Up against Foucault: Explorations of Some Tensions between Foucault and Feminism* (New York: Routledge, 1993) offers a collective reading more in line with Sawicki's critical engagement rather than MacDonald's or Levin's outright dismissal. Though still worth thinking about, the debates are not as fervent as they were in the early 1990s.

38. Alexandra Howson, "Embodied Obligation," 225, emphasis in original.
39. Alexandra Howson, "Embodied Obligation," 237.
40. She does mention femininity, but only in relation to citizenship and regulation in interpreting some of the women's feelings (226–28). She does not draw out the way in which the discourse about femininity actually manifests through social practices in health promotion and illness prevention.
41. David Wilson and Pamela Moss, "Spatiality Studies in Urban Geography," in *Research in Urban Sociology, vol. 4*, ed. Ray Hutchinson (Greenwich, Conn.: JAI Press, 1997), 5.

NOTES FOR CHAPTER 5

1. Clifford Geertz, *Local Knowledge* (New York: Basic, 1983), 10.
2. See discussion of reflexivity in the focus section on "Women in the Field," *Professional Geographer* 46 (1995): 54–102. See also Gillian Rose, "Situating Knowledges: Positionality, Reflexivities and Other Tactics," *Progress in Human Geography* 21 (1997): 305–20, who points out that we cannot know or fully understand all the aspects of the complex dynamics and processes of qualitative research. See also Isabel Dyck, Judith M. Lynam, and Joan M. Anderson, "Women Talking: Creating Knowledge through Difference in Cross-cultural Research," *Women's Studies International Forum* 18 (1995): 611–26; and Isabel Dyck and Arlene Tigar McLaren, "Telling It Like It Is . . . or Just Another Story? Tales of Immigrant Settlement." Unpublished manuscript available from first author at the School of Rehabilitations Sciences, University of British Columbia, Vancouver, BC, V6T 1B5, for specific

explorations within particular research projects. Joan Marshall, "Borderlands and Feminist Ethnography," in *Feminist Geography in Practice: Research and Methods*, ed. Pamela Moss (London: Blackwell, 2002), 174–86, discusses the difference between conversations and interviews in ethnographic work in a small island community.

3. We recognize that the academy does not value non-textual discursive spaces as contributions to the generation of knowledge. Yet methodological discussions, as frozen printed matter in the pages of academic journals, do not always encapsulate the texture of the social practices that produce and reproduce feminist research as a particular discourse (see Pamela Moss, "Opening Up Discursive Space for Engaging Reflexive Methods," presentation at the annual meeting of the Canadian Association of Geographers, St. Catharines, Ont., Canada, May 2000).

4. For an interesting discussion of this dynamic in-depth interviews, see Gill Valentine, "People Like Us: Negotiating Sameness and Difference in the Research Process," in *Feminist Geography in Practice*, 116–26.

5. Transcription itself involves some selection in itself—punctuation, spelling, inclusion or omission of sighs, laughter, pauses, and "uhms." Transcription also distances the analyst from the energy and synergy of the structured conversation of an interview. Transcripts are, in this way, disembodied. Analysts—who are not always the interviewers—rely on recall, field notes, and/or close discussion with the interviewer in an attempt to gain some of the texture of the embodied interview.

6. "Bibbet" is from Sandra Kirby and Kate McKenna, *Experience Research Social Change: Methods from the Margins* (Toronto: Garamond Press, 1989).

7. Donna Haraway, "Situated Knowledges: The Science Question in Feminism and the Privilege of Partial Perspective," *Feminist Studies* 14 (1998): 575–95, has been enormously influential in setting out the issues of the partiality of knowledge in her challenge of conventional notions of objectivity.

8. See Pamela Moss, "Negotiating Spaces in Home Environments: Older Women Living with Arthritis," *Social Science and Medicine* 45 (1997): 23–33.

9. She writes about these topics in: "Autobiographical Notes on Chronic Illness," *Mind and Body Spaces: Geographies of Illness, Impairment, and Disability*, ed. Ruth Butler and Hester Parr (New York: Routledge, 1999), 155–66; "Not Quite Abled, Not Quite Disabled: Experiences of Being 'In Between' ME and the Academy," *Disability Studies Quarterly* 20, no. 3 (2000): 287–93; and "Writing One's Life," in *Placing Autobiography in Geography*, ed. Pamela Moss (Syracuse, N.Y.: Syracuse University Press, 2001), 1–21.

10. See Pamela Moss and Margo Matwychuk, "Beyond Speaking as an 'As A' and Stating the 'Etc.' toward a Praxis of Difference," *Frontiers* 21, no. 3 (2000): 82–104; and Pamela Moss and Martha McMahon, "Between a Flake and a Strident Bitch: Making 'It' Count in the Academy," *Resources for Feminist Research/Documentation sur la recherche féministe* 28, nos. 1 and 2 (2000): 15–32, for how she uses insights gained from her experiences of illness and how these shaped her politics and analysis.

11. The study consisted of a first phase of semi-structured, in-depth interviewing of 54 women in different relationships to employment, who were recruited through a local branch of the Multiple Sclerosis Society and a city hospital. A questionnaire survey derived from dominant themes in the qualitative study followed, and was

completed by women recruited through a clinic directory. Co-investigator of the study was Dr. Lyn Jongbloed, whose expertise lies in policy analysis and quantitative methods. Results of this study and discussion of its methodology appear in a number of publications. Isabel Dyck, "Hidden Geographies: The Changing Lifeworlds of Women with Multiple Sclerosis," *Social Science and Medicine* 40 (1995): 307–20; "Whose Body? Whose Voice?" *Atlantis* 21 (1996): 54–62; "Women with Disabilities and Everyday Geographies: Home Space and the Contested Body," in *Putting Health into Place: Landscape, Identity and Wellbeing*, ed. Robin A. Kearns and Wil M. Gesler, 102–9 (Syracuse, N.Y.: Syracuse University Press, 1998); and "Body Troubles: Women, the Workplace, and Negotiations of a Disabled Identity," in *Mind and Body Spaces*, 119–37. See also Isabel Dyck and Lyn Jongbloed "Women with Multiple Sclerosis and Employment Issues: A Focus on Social and Institutional Environments," *Canadian Journal of Occupational Therapy* 67 (2000): 337–46; Lyn Jongbloed, "Factors Influencing Employment Status of Women with Multiple Sclerosis," *Canadian Journal of Rehabilitation* 9 (1996): 213–22; and Lyn Jongbloed, "Disability Income: The Experiences of Women with Multiple Sclerosis," *Canadian Journal of Occupational Therapy* 65 (1998): 193–201.

12. Pamela Moss and Isabel Dyck, "Inquiry into Environment and Body: Women, Work, and Chronic Illness," *Environment & Planning D: Society and Space* 14 (1996): 631–783.

13. For a more detailed discussion of these concerns in her research, see Isabel Dyck, "Putting Ethical Research into Practice: Issues of Context," *Ethics, Place and Environment* 3, no. 1 (2000): 80–87.

14. Pamela and Kathleen Gabelmann, graduate student and research assistant, conducted the interviews in Victoria. Kathleen, Isabel, and Ann Vanderbijl, research assistant, undertook the interviews in Vancouver.

15. The bulk of the interviews (41 of 48) were transcribed by two people, one of whom contracted out five of the interviews. One interview was transcribed by Monika Tvrdon, undergraduate research assistant. The remaining interview was transcribed by a community worker.

16. Note that we talked with the women only *after* the tenuous and unsettling process of obtaining a biomedically sound diagnosis of ME. Had we talked during the period of being unsettled, our analysis and theory would look different. We would anticipate that we would have focused primarily on fluctuating identities and legitimating bodily sensations. But, because we identified women on the basis of a biomedical diagnosis, we were able to solicit accounts of approaches to treatment and struggles over disability claims.

17. Most of the women in the study used ME denoting their illness. In Canada and the U.K., ME is favored by advocacy groups because of the legitimacy such a complex name gives the biomedical and popular community. Leonard A. Jason, Renee R. Taylor, Zuzana Stepanek, and Sigita Pliopys, in "Attitudes Regarding Chronic Fatigue Syndrome: The Importance of a Name," *Journal of Health Psychology* 6, no. 1 (2001): 61–71, give support to this claim. They found that interns and residents in a Chicago area hospital were more likely to diagnose ME in lieu of two other names referring to the *same* constellation of symptoms—Chronic Fatigue and Immune Dysfunction Syndrome (CFIDS) and Florence Nightingale Disease.

18. See Anthony L. Komaroff and Laura R. Fagioli, "Medical Assessment of Fatigue and Chronic Fatigue Syndrome," in *Chronic Fatigue Syndrome: An Integrative Approach to Evaluation and Treatment*, ed. Mark A. Dematrack and Susan E. Abbey, 154–80 (New York: Guilford, 1996).

19. The simplicity of this test to indicate RA is being challenged. Malcolm L. Bridgen in "Clinical Utility of the Erythrocyte Sedimentation Rate," *American Family Physician* October (1999): 1443–54, argues that without evidence of other symptoms, the ESR should not be used as the only indicator of disease.

20. This does not mean that women with RA have an "easier" time legitimating their illness socially. Biomedically, there may be acceptance, but this works in the women's favor only occasionally. Women with RA still face disbelief and neglect among friends, family members, and strangers.

21. This project was funded through the Canadian Aging Research Network (CARNET; principal investigator, Neena Chappell) through the Centre on Aging, University of Victoria. Pamela's project consisted of in-depth interviews with 23 women, ranging in age from 62 to 93 and three men, from 72 to 84.

22. For the project, Pamela was primarily responsible for the conceptual development, analysis, and writing for the project, including what is presented in this book.

23. We decided not to provide any in-depth analysis of class position, race, ethnicity, or sexuality, not because we do not think them important; rather, we want to focus on the instability of identity, destabilization of materiality, and the spatiality of everyday life through the context of chronic illness, specifically ME and RA.

Although most of the women, especially with ME, appear to be professionals and homeowners with middle-range incomes, this should not be read as supporting stereotypes of which women develop ME. Studies undertaken at DePaul University show that ME is not a "yuppie disease." Leonard A. Jason, Judith A. Richman, Alfred W. Rademaker, Karen M. Jordon, Audrius V. Plioplys, Renee R. Taylor, William McCready, Cheng-Fang Huang, and Sigita Plioplys, "A Community-based Study of Chronic Fatigue Syndrome," *Archives of Internal Medicine (JAMA)* 159, no. 18 (October 11, 1999) [http//archinte.ama-assn.org/issues/v159n18/full/ioi90161.html], argue that prevalence rates are just as high among older adults as they are among younger adults and that rates may be higher among visible minority groups and lower income people. They explain this discrepancy in incidence reporting by citing limited access to medical care as the leading cause of not being diagnosed. Many poorer people with debilitating fatigue drop out of the health care system and have no way of showing up in the health service statistics. Along these same lines, this high incidence of home ownership is also probably not indicative of women in general or women with chronic illness in particular.

NOTES FOR CHAPTER 6

1. For a more detailed discussion of this legitimation process for women diagnosed with chronic illness, see Pamela Moss and Isabel Dyck, "Body, Corporeal Space, and Legitimating Chronic Illness: Women Diagnosed with M.E.," *Antipode* 31 (1999): 371–97. Susan Wendell in *The Rejected Body* (New York: Routledge,

1996) notes the importance of social and cognitive authority of biomedicine in legitimizing her illness (ME), without which her symptoms remained invalidated.

2. *Shigella* [bacteria] spreads rapidly through inadequately treated drinking
water that can be the result of low reserves, untreated sewage, or loose charcoal filter
beds.

3. Reiter's Syndrome is a systemic rheumatic disease involving the inflammation
of joints, eyes (conjunctivitis), mouth lining, aorta, and urinary, genital, or gastrointestinal systems. Shigella virus is known to activate the syndrome.

4. As described by Elizabeth Grosz, "Bodies and Knowledges: Feminism and
the Crisis of Reason," in *Space, Time, and Perversion* (New York: Routledge, 1995),
32–38.

5. Because of her own experiences of chronic illness, Vivienne thinks that her
mother actually had ME, but was never diagnosed.

6. Pamela discusses her own experiences with ME in "Autobiographical Notes
on Chronic Illness," in *Mind and Body Spaces: Geographies of Disability, Illness, and
Impairment*, ed. Ruth Butler and Hester Parr, 155–66 (New York: Routledge, 1999)
and "Not Quite Abled and Not Quite Disabled: Experiences of Being 'In Between'
ME and the Academy," *Disability Studies Quarterly* 20, vol. 3 (2000): 287–93.

7. Abigail Bray and Claire Colebrook, "The Haunted Flesh: Corporeal Feminism and the Politics of (Dis)Embodiment," *Signs* 24, no. 1 (1998): 57.

8. Grosz, "Bodies and Knowledges," 36.

9. Claire Colebrook, in "Feminist and Autonomy: The Crisis of the Self-
Authoring Subject," *Body and Society* 3, no. 2 (1997): 21–41, suggest that the concept of autonomy needs to be reworked. In critiquing modernist thinking, she
argues that autonomy can be conceived through the body so that there is no fixed
position for the subject to follow: "The body is not just a condition or limit to
thought, it is rather the medium through which the relation to the other takes place.
Autonomy is no longer formal self-legislation, no longer a process of abstraction or
negation; it is now defined as the specific sense of embodiment given through the
relation to the embodied other" (39).

NOTES FOR CHAPTER 7

1. We have, in the past, problematized the concept of environment in Pamela
Moss and Isabel Dyck, "Inquiry into Environment and Body: Women, Work, and
Chronic Illness," *Environment and Planning D: Society and Space* 14 (1996): 746.

By casting environment as socially negotiated space inclusive of its material
aspects we can get beyond experientially based, individualistic, humanist conceptions of place as well as incorporating hegemonically defined notions of particular environments. Environment is embedded in a socially constructed space
that acts as a medium of social relations discursively shaping and reshaping
both individuals and places. Conceptualizing environment solely in discursive
terms, however, does not recognise privileged positions of power nor the ability
of individuals to resist processes structuring space. Explicit recognition of
uneven distributions of privileged power positions and the material conditions

of existence is needed in order to circumscribe the power within the social relations that shape and reshape environment. Within this circumscription of
power, it is necessary to conceive boundaries of environment as shifting entities
that continuously expand and shrink, are negotiated and renegotiated, and are
constantly being drawn and redrawn, in accordance with those relations that
(re)structure that environment.

This more complex notion of environment still holds in our work here. We
would, however, emphasize and try to draw out more clearly, the constitutive aspects
of processes structuring space. And, perhaps rather than discussing "uneven distributions of privileged power positions," we would discuss the highly textured arrangements of particularized deployments of power.

2. These "failings" are evident in the prevalence of diagnosing women, at the
turn of the last century, with Neurasthenia and, in the last quarter of the past century, with depression. A commonsense response to personal "failing" would be to
work on personal development in an attempt to become a "better person."

3. This harkens back to Armando Favazza's work about self-mutilation and
Fakir Musafar's critique about states of grace (Armando R. Favazza, *Bodies under
Siege: Self-Mutilation and Body Modification in Culture and Psychiatry,* Baltimore:
Johns Hopkins University Press, 1996; and Fakir Musafar, "Body Play: State of
Grace or Sickness?" in *Bodies under Siege,* 325–34) that we discussed in chapter 3.
Instead of marking themselves physically or seeking out pain, these women, already
marked and in pain, seek a "state of grace" as a way to deal with the intensity of
their material body.

4. An interesting contrast to Belle's destabilization is Sandy Slack's discussion
of her experiences of being in/using a wheelchair in "I Am More Than My Wheels,"
in *Disability and Discourse,* ed. Marian Corker and Sally French, 28–38 (London:
Open University Press, 1999). Slack focuses on the constitution of her identity as a
disabled woman through her use of an old style, heavy, privately owned wheelchair
and her use of a new, lightweight, state-owned one that she has because of her
employment.

5. Fred Friedberg and Leonard A. Jason in *Understanding Chronic Fatigue Syndrome: An Empirical Guide to Assessment and Treatment* (Washington: American Psychological Association, 2000) begin from this point of rejection to build a
framework for psychiatrists, psychologists, and physicians to use as a departure point
for understanding the physicality of the illness in conjunction with the psychological
aspects of the disease.

6. See Emily Martin, *Flexible Bodies: The Role of Immunity in American Culture
from the Days of Polio to the Age of AIDS* (Boston: Beacon Press, 1994). Martin
argues that using the metaphor of the immune system as a fortress has shaped the
social practices of biomedicine.

7. We use this as a reference to a video, "Beyond These Four Walls," produced
by Kari Krogh and the Home Support Action Group in Victoria, Canada, as part
of a participatory action research project. In the video, recipients of home support
protest cuts in home care by drawing on their own experience. The video is being
used to lobby the government to stop cutting and to restore funding for home support and raise consciousness about the issue among the general public and specific

groups who are also facing reduced health care services. The video and the accompanying report is available through http://www.ryerson.ca/~kkrogh/report1/toc.html.

8. See Edward H. Yelin, "Gender, Disability, and Employment," *Occupational Medicine* 8 (1993): 849–58; Lyn Jongbloed, "Factors Influencing Employment Status of Women with Multiple Sclerosis," *Canadian Journal of Rehabilitation* 9 (1996): 213–22; Isabel Dyck, "Body Troubles: Women, the Workplace, and Negotiations of a Disabled Identity," in *Mind and Body Spaces: Geographies of Illness, Impairment and Disability,* ed. Ruth Butler and Hester Parr, 119–37 (New York: Routledge, 1999); Carolyn S. Dewa and Elizabeth Lin, "Chronic Physical Illness, Psychiatric Disorder and Disability in the Workplace," *Social Science & Medicine* 51 (2000): 41–50; and Julia Faucett, Paul D. Blanc, and Edward H. Yelin, "The Impact of Carpal Tunnel Syndrome on Work Status: Implications of Job Characteristics for Staying on the Job," *Journal of Occupational Rehabilitation* 10, no. 1 (2000): 55–69.

9. See for example, Carolyn Vash, "Employment Issues for Women with Disabilities," *Rehabilitation Literature* 43, nos. 7 and 8 (1982): 198–207; Freda L. Paltiel "The Disabled Women's Network in Canada," *Sexuality and Disability* 5, no. 1 (1997): 47–50; and Gail Fawcett, in *Bringing Down the Barriers: The Labour Market and Women with Disabilities in Ontario* (Ottawa: Canadian Council on Social Development, 2000).

10. Sometimes this is referred to as a "double handicap" in the literature, see Mary Jo Deegan and Nancy A. Brooks, *Women and Disability: The Double Handicap* (New Brunswick, N.J.: Transaction, 1985).

11. Elaine Brody, " 'Women in the Middle' and Family Help to Older People," *The Gerontologist* 21 (1981): 471–80; Jane Lewis and Barbara Meredith, *Daughters Who Care: Daughters Caring for Mothers at Home* (London: Routledge & Kegan Paul, 1988); Baila Miller, "Gender Differences in Spouse Management of the Caregiver Role," in *Circles of Care: Work and Identity in Women's Lives,* ed. Emily K. Abel and Margaret K. Nelson, 92–104 (New York: SUNY Press, 1990); and Judy Singleton, "Women Caring for Elderly Family Members: Shaping Non-traditional Work and Family Initiatives," *Journal of Comparative Family Studies* 31 (2000): 367–75.

12. See Patricia Kolb, "Continuing to Care: Black and Latina Daughters' Assistance to Their Mothers in Nursing Homes," *Affilia* 15 (2000): 502–25; and Cathy D. Martin, "More Than the Work: Race and Gender Differences in Caregiving Burden," *Journal of Family Issues* 21 (2000): 986–1005.

13. See in particular Jane Aronson, "Dutiful Daughters and Undemanding Mothers: Constraining Images of Giving and Receiving Care in Middle and Later Life," in *Women's Caring: Feminist Perspectives on Social Welfare,* 2nd ed., ed. Carol Baines, Patricia Evans and Sheila Neysmith, 114–38 (Toronto: Oxford University Press, 1998); and Gillian Dalley, *Ideologies of Caring: Rethinking Community and Collectivism* (Basingstoke, U.K.: Macmillan Education in association with the Centre for Policy on Ageing, 1996 [1988]).

14. Several examples exist that draw on the perspectives of "patients" in order to understand the impact of chronic illness on women's lives. Examples include Ruth Pinder, "Striking Balances: Living with Parkinson's Disease," in *Living with Chronic*

Illness: The Experiences of Patients and their Families, ed. Robert Anderson and Michael Bury, 67–88 (London: Hyman Unwin, 1988); Jenny Strong, Roderick Ashton, David Chant, and Tess Cramond, "An Investigation of the Dimensions of Chronic Low Back Pain: The Patients' Perspectives," *British Journal of Occupational Therapy* 57 (1994): 204–8; Chris M. Henriksson, "Living with Continuous Muscular Pain—Patient Perspectives, Part 1: Encounters and Consequences," *Scandinavian Journal of Caring Science* 9 (1995): 67–76; and Nancy G. Klimas and Roberto Patarca, eds., *Disability and Chronic Fatigue Syndrome: Clinical, Legal and Patient Perspectives* (New York: Haworth Press, 1997).

15. Julia was successful in this strategy. But in an ironic twist of fate, as soon as she could declare herself recovered from ME, she was laid off due to restructuring. For more details of Julia's story, see Pamela Moss and Isabel Dyck, "Material Bodies Precariously Positioned: Women Embodying Chronic Illness in the Workplace," in *Geographies of Women's Health*, ed. Isabel Dyck, Nancy Davis Lewis, and Sara McLafferty, 235–37 (New York: Routledge, 2001), and for Sandra's, 240–41.

16. Debbie Leslie and David Butz make this point in " 'GM Suicide': Flexibility, Space, and the Injured Body," *Economic Geography* 74 (1998): 360–78. They argue that economic restructuring takes place at a number of scales, including the body by setting up them up as vulnerable to injuries through an imposition an unfamiliar set of material and discursive practices.

17. Reann then went on sick leave again and secured income from a state pension and private long-term disability.

18. This harkens back to Ruth Pinder's argument in "Sick-but-fit or Fit-but-sick? Ambiguity and Identity in the Workplace," in *Exploring the Divide: Illness and Disability*, ed. Colin Barnes and Geoff Mercer, 135–56 (Leeds, U.K.: Disability Press, 1996).

19. Margrit Shildrick and Janet Price in "Breaking the Boundaries of the Broken Body," *Body and Society* 2, no. 4 (1996): 93–113.

20. On many forms there is a question that addresses this issue generally. It is often phrased as post-exercise exertion and counted in terms of days.

21. "Serial sevens" involves the person being tested to begin with 100 and count backwards by seven. In "walking a line heel-toe," a person walks the length of an doctor's office on an imaginary line with each step comprised of a heel touching a toe. The "tilt-table test" is a protocol designed to measure blood pressure and pulse at a 70-degree tilt for one minute, and thereafter every five minutes. This test is repeated if the person being tested can tolerate the tilt. In all these tests, physicians are trying to determine neurological functioning and impairment.

22. We discuss in more depth this process of appropriating discursive categories rooted in one discourse and developing a set of social practices associated with a different discourse in Pamela Moss and Isabel Dyck, "Body, Corporeal Space and Legitimating Chronic Illness: Women Diagnosed with ME," *Antipode* 31 (1999): 372–97.

23. We purposefully do not identify this woman.

24. Titles of books emphasize fluidity and permeability: Margrit Shildrick, *Leaky Bodies and Boundaries: Feminism, Postmodernism and (Bio)Ethics* (New York: Routledge, 1997) and Robyn Longhurst, *Bodies: Exploring Fluid Boundaries* (New York: Routledge, 2001).

NOTES FOR CHAPTER 8

1. See our discussion about Chantal Mouffe and nodal points in chapter 1.

2. In an informal telephone survey of 11 insurance companies issuing life insurance policies for people with ME, MS, cancer, and HIV in Capital Region District (CRD), including 17 municipalities on southern Vancouver Island in spring 1998, we found that people with HIV were most likely to get refused, then ME, MS, and cancer in that order. Of the 11, one company was cautious and did not reveal any criteria for issuing policies for people with chronic illness. Eight representatives claimed the company would refuse people with HIV, while one company would accept people with HIV if they were in a group plan at discovery, and an additional company deferred to answer questions about HIV. For people with cancer, all ten life insurance companies would issue policies depending on the type of cancer, severity, and status of remission. Nine companies would also issue policies for people with MS with the only variable being severity. One agent said that it would be doubtful to insure anyone with MS. Questions about ME produced complex results, which is not surprising given the contested status of the disease. Criteria for issuing a policy varied: dependent on the status of individual prognosis; would be a possibility as long as there is not another variable involved with the example given as breast cancer; will not issue if within two years of diagnosis because of suicide threat; will issue as long as ME is not life-threatening with severity measured by medication prescribed; and needing to know if the problem could be fixed through, for example, surgery. No representative was willing to claim that the company would issue a policy to someone diagnosed with ME; all were cautious citing higher rates and vague possibilities of coverage with the need to do more research. Three agents noted that giving life insurance to a person with ME would be like purchasing fire insurance when the building was on fire. One of these agents went on further to say that insurance is really about "healthy" people and that "healthy" people wanted a "healthy" pool of people to be part of their money investment. Group insurance is for people who are ill.

What we can draw out of this survey is that ME is scrutinized more closely than the other three illnesses. Rheumatoid arthritis was not an issue with any of these insurance companies. For illnesses that have been more medicalized, like cancer and HIV, there are clearer protocols for issuing life insurance. Among insurance providers, there seems to be an acceptance that there exists a wide variation in how ME and MS play out as illnesses. However, the information in this survey indicates that MS is a bit more legitimate than ME. That Reann said, "you can't get life insurance" demonstrates the popularized knowledge circulating about ME possibly causing difficulties in future financial security.

As a final, anecdotal note on this topic, by fall 1999, one of these insurance companies, a company where one of the agents used the analogy of the building being on fire, had changed the parameters of applying for group life insurance. On the application, a question determining whether the applicant had ever been diagnosed with Chronic Fatigue Syndrome (CFS) was included as a possibility for outright denial.

3. Although she does refer to being "useful," we think her point here is to resist

inscriptions of dominant discourses that would define her as a woman and as a woman with chronic illness.

4. Recall that these activities are ones they engage as part of the process of the formation of self (see Abigail Bray and Claire Colebrook, "The Haunted Flesh: Corporeal Feminism and the Politics of (Dis)Embodiment," *Signs* 24, no. 1 (1998): 35–67).

5. For a description of possible barriers lesbian women face in the disability community and disabled women face in the lesbian community, see Ruth Butler, "Double the Trouble or Twice the Fun? Disabled Bodies in the Gay Community," in *Mind and Body Spaces: Geographies of Illness, Impairment and Disability*, ed. Ruth Butler and Hester Parr, 203–20 (New York: Routledge, 1999).

6. Like most other chronic illness, women access knowledge and resources about ME through newsletters, electronic newsgroups, web sites, and books. For example, most groups have newsletters and/or web sites (see http://members.home.com/me.victoria/). The ME/FM Action Network in Ottawa lobbies Parliament on behalf of women with ME and Fibromyalgia Syndrome (http://www3.sympatico.ca/me-fm.action/). Co-Cure, or "Co-operate and Communicate for a Cure, (www.co-cure.org) circulates news items and research about ME and FMS by e-mail. The Co-Cure archives can be found at http://listserv.nodak.edu/archives/co-cure.html. The U.S. national organization, CFIDS Association of America (www.cfids.org) is a well-organized and high-profile advocacy group that provides resources and references on-line. There are several introductory books on the treatment and assessment of ME that women may find useful, including Erica F. Verillo and Lauren M. Gellman, *Chronic Fatigue Syndrome: A Treatment Guide* (New York: Quality Medical Publishing, 1998) and Fred Friedberg and Leonard A. Jason, in *Understanding Chronic Fatigue Syndrome: An Empirical Guide to Assessment and Treatment* (Washington: American Psychological Association, 2000).

7. Hillary Johnson, *Osler's Web: Inside the Labyrinth of the Chronic Fatigue Syndrome Epidemic* (New York: Crown, 1996).

8. This is not entirely true. Women with ME often have glazed eyes, awkward movements, and drawn facial features. The gait is sometimes uneven as is balance.

NOTES FOR CHAPTER 9

1. These proclamations or dismissals have varying effects on ill women. Research outside the Foucauldian tradition has focused on the interaction between time and space, and has found that women's and community health clinics have empowering effects. See, for example, Megan Warin, Frances Baum, Elizabeth Kalucy, Charlie Murray, and Bronwyn Veale, "The Power of Place: Space and Time in Women's and Community health Centres in South Australia," *Social Science and Medicine* 50 (2000): 1863–75.

2. This interaction is quite complex for women (and men) when presenting with symptoms associated with ME. Jonathan Banks and Lindsay Prior, "Doing Things with Illness: The Micro Politics of the CFS Clinic," *Social Science and Medicine* 52 (2001): 11–23, describe the process through physicians and patients in the

United Kingdom negotiate the diagnosis of ME. They examine how competing knowledges play out in the clinical interview. Physicians primarily follow the biomedical guidelines set out for diagnosis in the Joint Working Group on CFS (Chronic Fatigue Syndrome), whereas patients tend to follow the position of the ME/CFS Alliance. The former views CFS (refusing the label of ME) as both a social and psychological disorder, whereas the latter claims that ME (the preferred label) is an organic condition. They show that these clinical encounters are contests wherein both physician and patient continually demarcate and redefine the boundaries between mind and body through manifestations between psychology and pathology.

3. Methodologically, we relied on volunteers to be part of the study. We did not turn anyone away. It happened that the women with ME all had been diagnosed by either a biomedical or naturopathic physician. Regarding the women with arthritis, all had severe RA with one woman also having Ankylosing Spondylitis. However, the onset varied—Belle, Carolyn, Margie, and Ronnie had onset as children; onset for the rest was as adults.

NOTES FOR CHAPTER 10

1. Joan W. Scott, " 'Experience,' " in *Feminists Theorize the Political*, ed. Judith Butler and Joan W. Scott (New York: Routledge, 1992).

2. See, for example, Rosemary Hennessy and Chrys Ingraham, eds., *Materialist Feminism: A Reader in Class, Difference, and Women's Lives* (New York: Routledge, 1995); and Theresa Ebert, *Ludic Feminism and After: Postmodernism, Desire, and Labor in Late Capitalism* (Ann Arbor: University of Michigan Press, 1996).

3. Racialized women with chronic illness rarely appear in the literature. See, however, Joan M. Anderson, Connie Blue, and A. Lau, "Women's Perspectives on Chronic Illness: Ethnicity, Ideology, and Restructuring of Life," *Social Science and Medicine* 33 (1991): 101–13; Nasa Begum, "Disabled Women and the Feminist Agenda," *Feminist Review* 40 (1992): 3–6; and Nasa Begum, "Doctor, Doctor . . . Disabled Women's Experiences of General Practitioners," in *Encounters with Strangers: Feminism and Disability*, ed. Jenny Morris (London: Women's Press, 1996), 168–93; and Isabel Dyck, "Putting Chronic Illness 'In Place': Women Immigrants' Account of their Health Care," *Geoforum* 26, no. 3 (1995): 247–60.

4. Although we did not set out to choose women based on sexuality, there were several women in the study who self-identified as lesbian.

5. We want to emphasize that we are not conflating citizenship and race. We recognize these as separate conceptualizations.

Bibliography

Abbey, Susan E., and Paul E. Garfinkel. "Neurasthenia and Chronic Fatigue Syndrome: The Role of Culture in the Making of a Diagnosis." *American Journal of Psychiatry* 148, no. 12 (December 1991): 1638–46.

Ainley, Rosa, ed. *New Frontiers of Space, Bodies, and Gender.* New York: Routledge, 1998.

Anderson, Joan M., Connie Blue, and A. Lau. "Women's Perspectives on Chronic Illness: Ethnicity, Ideology and Restructuring of Life." *Social Science and Medicine* 33 (1991): 101–13

Anderson, Vivienne. "A Will of Its Own: Experiencing the Body in Severe Chronic Illness." In *Women's Bodies/Women's Lives: Health, Well-Being, and Body Image*, ed. Baukje Miedema, Janet M. Stoppard, and Vivienne Anderson. Toronto: Sumach Press, 2000.

Aronson, Jane. "Dutiful Daughters and Undemanding Mothers: Constraining Images of Giving and Receiving Care in Middle and Later Life." In *Women's Caring: Feminist Perspectives on Social Welfare.* 2nd ed, ed. Carol Baines, Patricia Evans, and Sheila Neysmith. Toronto: Oxford University Press, 1998.

Banks, Jonathan, and Lindsay Prior. "Doing Things with Illness: The Micro Politics of the CFS Clinic." *Social Science and Medicine* 52 (2001): 11–23.

Barnes, Trevor, and James Duncan, eds. *Writing Worlds: Discourse, Text, and Metaphor in the Representation of Landscape.* New York: Routledge, 1992.

Begum, Nasa. "Disabled Women and the Feminist Agenda." *Feminist Review* 40 (1992): 3–6.

———. "Doctor, Doctor . . . Disabled Women's Experiences of General Practitioners." In *Encounters with Strangers: Feminism and Disability*, ed. Jenny Morris, 168–93. London: Women's Press, 1996.

Bell, David, Jon Binnie, Julia Cream, and Gill Valentine. "All Hyped Up and No Place to Go." *Gender, Place & Culture* 1 (1994): 31–48.

Bell, David, and Gill Valentine, eds. *Maps of Desire.* New York: Routledge, 1995.

Benhabib, Seyla. "The Generalized and the Concrete Other: The Kohlberg-Gilligan Controversy and Moral Theory." In *Situating the Self: Gender, Community, and Postmodernism in Contemporary Ethics.* New York: Routledge, 1992.

Benner, Patricia. "The Roles of Embodiment, Emotion, and Lifeworld for Rationality and Agency in Nursing Practice." *Nursing Philosophy* 1, no. 1 (2000): 5–19.

————, ed. *Interpretive Phenomenology: Embodiment, Caring, and Ethics in Health and Illness.* Thousand Oaks, Calif.: Sage, 1994.

Blecher, Mark J. "The Shaping of Psychoanalytic Theory and Practice." In *Disorienting Sexuality: Psychoanalytic Reappraisals of Sexual Identities,* ed. Thomas Domenici and Ronnie C. Lesser. New York: Routledge, 1995.

Blunt, Alison, and Jane Wills. "Embodying Geography: Feminist Geographies of Gender." In *Dissident Geographies: An Introduction to Radical Ideas and Practice.* Harlow: Longman, 2000.

Bondi, Liz. "Locating Identity Politics." In *Place and the Politics of Identity,* ed. Michael Keith and Steve Pile. New York: Routledge, 1993.

————. "Stages on Journeys: Some Remarks about Human Geography and Psychotherapeutic Practice." *Professional Geographer* 51 (1999): 11–24.

Bordo, Susan. *Unbearable Weight: Feminism, Western Culture, and the Body.* Berkeley: University of California Press, 1993.

Boston Women's Health Book Collective, *Our Bodies, Ourselves: A Book by and for Women.* New York: Simon and Schuster, 1972.

————. *Our Bodies, Ourselves: A Book by and for Women.* New York: Simon and Schuster, 1992.

Bourdieu, Pierre. *Outline of a Theory of Practice.* Cambridge: Cambridge University Press, 1977.

Bray, Abigail, and Claire Colebrook. "The Haunted Flesh: Corporeal Feminism and the Politics of (Dis)Embodiment." *Signs* 24, no. 1 (1998): 35–67.

Bridgen, Malcolm L. "Clinical Utility of the Erythrocyte Sedimentation Rate." *American Family Physician* (October 1999): 1443–54.

Brody, Elaine. " 'Women in the Middle' and Family Help to Older People." *The Gerontologist* 21 (1981): 471–80.

Bury, Michael. "Chronic Illness as Biographical Disruption." *Sociology of Health and Illness* 4, no. 2 (1982): 167–82.

Butler, Judith. "Foucault and the Paradox of Bodily Inscriptions." *The Journal of Philosophy* 86, no. 11 (1989): 601–7.

————. *Gender Trouble: Feminism and the Subversion of Identity.* New York: Routledge, 1990.

————. *Bodies That Matter: On the Discursive Limits of "Sex."* New York: Routledge, 1993.

————. *Excitable Speech: A Politics of the Performative.* New York: Routledge, 1997.

Butler, Ruth. "Double the Trouble or Twice the Fun? Disabled Bodies in the Gay Community." In *Mind and Body Spaces: Geographies of Illness, Impairment, and Disability,* ed. Ruth Butler and Hester Parr. New York: Routledge, 1999.

Butler, Ruth, and Sophia Bowlby. "Bodies and Spaces: An Exploration of Disabled People's Experiences of Public Space." *Environment and Planning D: Society and Space* 15 (1997): 411–33.

Butler, Ruth, and Hester Parr, eds. *Mind and Body Spaces: Geographies of Illness, Impairment, and Disability.* New York: Routledge, 1999.

Callard, Felicity J. "The Body in Theory." *Environment & Planning D: Society & Space* 16 (1998): 387–400.

Charmaz, Kathy. *Good Days, Bad Days.* New Brunswick, N.J.: Rutgers University Press, 1991.

Chouinard, Vera, and Ali Grant. "On Not Being Anywhere Near the 'Project.' " *Antipode* 27 (1995): 137–66.

Cixous, Hélène. "Castration or Decapitation?" *Signs* 7 (1981): 41–55.

Cixous, Hélène, and Catherine Clément. *The Newly Born Woman*, trans. Betsy Wing. Minneapolis: University of Minnesota Press, 1986.

Cockburn, Cynthia. *Brothers: Male Dominance and Technological Change.* London: Pluto Press, 1990.

Colebrook, Claire. "Feminist and Autonomy: The Crisis of the Self-Authoring Subject." *Body and Society* 3, no. 2 (1997): 21–41.

Comacchio, Cynthia R. "Motherhood in Crisis: Women, Medicine, and State in Canada 1900–1940." In *Materialist Feminism: A Reader in Class, Difference, and Women's Lives*, ed. Rosemary Hennessy and Chrys Ingraham. New York: Routledge, 1995.

Cooper, Lesley, and Martin Walker. "Whose Hysteria?" *Continuum* 5, no. 1 (1997): 4–5.

Cream, Julia. "Women on Trial? A Private Pillory?" In *Mapping the Subject: Geographies of Cultural Transformation*, ed. Steve Pile and Nigel Thrift. New York: Routledge, 1995.

Crompton, Rosemary, and Kay Sanderson. *Gendered Jobs and Social Change.* London: Unwin Hyman, 1990.

Csordas, Thomas J., ed. *Embodiment and Experience: The Existential Ground of Culture and Self.* New York: Cambridge University Press, 1994.

Dalley, Gillian. *Ideologies of Caring: Rethinking Community and Collectivism.* Basingstoke, U.K.: Macmillan Education in association with the Centre for Policy on Aging, 1996 [1988].

Davidson, Joyce. "Fear and Trembling in the Mall: Women, Agoraphobia, and Body Boundaries." In *Geographies of Women's Health*, ed. Isabel Dyck, Nancy Davis Lewis, and Sara McLafferty. New York: Routledge, 2001.

Davis, Angela. *Women, Race, and Class.* New York: Random House, 1981.

Davis, Kathy. *Reshaping the Female Body: The Dilemma of Cosmetic Surgery.* New York: Routledge, 1995.

Deegan, Mary Jo, and Nancy A. Brooks. *Women and Disability: The Double Handicap.* New Brunswick, N.J.: Transaction Books, 1985.

Delaney, David, and Helga Leitner. "The Political Construction of Scale." *Political Geography* 16, no. 2 (1997): 93–97.

Deleuze, Gilles. *Difference and Repetition.* Trans. Paul Patton. New York: Columbia University, 1994.

Deleuze, Gilles, and Félix Guattari. *A Thousand Plateaus.* Minneapolis: University of Minnesota Press, 1987.

Derrida, Jacques. "Plato's Pharmacy." In *Dissemination*, trans. Barbara Johnson. Chicago: University of Chicago Press, 1981.

Dewa, Carolyn S., and Elizabeth Lin. "Chronic Physical Illness, Psychiatric Disorder and Disability in the Workplace." *Social Science & Medicine* 51 (2000): 41–50.

Diprose, Rosalyn. *The Bodies of Women: Ethics, Embodiment, and Sexual Difference.* New York: Routledge, 1993.

Domenici, Thomas, and Ronnie C. Lesser, eds. *Disorienting Sexuality: Psychoanalytic Reappraisals of Sexual Identities.* New York: Routledge, 1995.

Donchin, Anne, and Laura Martha Purdy. *Embodying Bioethics: Recent Feminist Advances.* Lanham, Md.: Rowman & Littlefield, 1999.

Dorn, Michael. "Beyond Nomadism: The Travel Narratives of a 'Cripple.' " In *Places through the Body,* ed. Heidi J. Nast and Steve Pile. New York: Routledge, 1998.

Dorn, Michael, and Glenda Laws. "Social Theory, Body Politics, and Medical Geography: Extending Kearns's Invitation." *Professional Geographer* 46, no. 1 (1994): 106–10.

Douglas, Mary. *Natural Symbols: Explorations in Cosmology.* London: Cresset Press, 1970.

Duff, Kat. *The Alchemy of Illness.* London: Virago, 1994.

Duncan, Nancy, ed. *Body/Space: Destabilizing Geographies of Gender and Sexuality.* New York: Routledge, 1996.

Dyck, Isabel. "Hidden Geographies: The Changing Lifeworlds of Women with Disabilities." *Social Science and Medicine* 40 (1995): 307–20

———. "Putting Chronic Illness 'In Place': Women Immigrants' Accounts of Their Health Care." *Geoforum* 26, no. 3 (1995): 247–60.

———. "Whose Body? Whose Voice?" *Atlantis* 21 (1996): 54–62.

———. "Body Troubles: Women, the Workplace, and Negotiations of a Disabled Identity." In *Mind and Body Spaces: Geographies of Illness, Impairment, and Disability,* ed. Ruth Butler and Hester Parr. New York: Routledge, 1999.

———. "Women with Disabilities and Everyday Geographies: Home, Space, and the Contested Body." In *Putting Health into Place: Landscape, Identity, and Wellbeing,* ed. Robin A. Kearns and Wil Gesler. Syracuse, N.Y.: Syracuse Press, 1998.

———. "Putting Ethical Research into Practice: Issues of Context." *Ethics, Place, and Environment* 3, no. 1 (2000): 80–87.

Dyck, Isabel, and Lyn Jongbloed. "Women with Multiple Sclerosis and Employment Issues: A Focus on Social and Institutional Environments." *Canadian Journal of Occupational Therapy* 67 (2000): 337–46.

Dyck, Isabel, Judith M. Lynam, and Joan M. Anderson. "Women Talking: Creating Knowledge through Difference in Cross-cultural Research." *Women's Studies International Forum* 18 (1995): 611–26.

Dyck, Isabel, and Arlene Tigar McLaren. "Telling It Like It Is . . . or Just Another Story? Tales of Immigrant Settlement." Unpublished manuscript available from first author at the School of Rehabilitations Sciences, University of British Columbia, Vancouver, BC, V6T 1B5.

Dyck, Isabel, Nancy Davis Lewis, and Sara McLafferty, eds. *Geographies of Women's Health.* New York: Routledge, 2001.

Ebert, Theresa. *Ludic Feminism and After: Postmodernism, Desire, and Labor in Late Capitalism.* Ann Arbor: University of Michigan Press, 1996.

Edelman, Lee. "The Plague of Discourse: Politics, Literary Theory, and AIDS." In *The Postmodern Turn: New Perspectives on Social Theory,* ed. Steven Seidman, 299–312. Cambridge: Cambridge University Press, 1994.

Elias, Norbert. *State Formation and Civilization.* Vol. 2 of *The Civilizing Process.* Oxford: Basil Blackwell, 1982 [1939].

Eyles, John. "From Disease Ecology and Spatial Analysis To . . . ? The Challenges of Medical Geography in Canada." *Health and Canadian Society* 1 (1993): 113–45.

Ezzy, Douglas. "Lived Experience and Interpretation in Narrative Theory: Experience of Living with HIV/AIDS." *Qualitative Sociology* 21 (1998): 169–80.

———. "Illness Narratives: Time, Hope and HIV." *Social Science and Medicine* 50 (2000): 605–17.

Fairhurst, Eileen. " 'Growing Old Gracefully' as Opposed to 'Mutton Dressed as Lamb': The Social Construction of Recognising Older Women." In *The Body in Everyday Life*, ed. Sarah Nettleton and Jonathan Watson. New York: Routledge, 1997.

Faucett, Julia, Paul D. Blanc, and Edward H. Yelin, "The Impact of Carpal Tunnel Syndrome on Work Status: Implications of Job Characteristics for Staying on the Job." *Journal of Occupational Rehabilitation* 10, no. 1 (2000): 55–69.

Favazza, Armando R. *Bodies under Siege: Self-Mutilation and Body Modification in Culture and Psychiatry*. Baltimore, Md.: Johns Hopkins University Press, 1996.

Fawcett, Gail. *Bringing Down the Barriers: The Labour Market and Women with Disabilities in Ontario*. Ottawa: Canadian Council on Social Development, 2000.

Ferguson, Anne. *Blood at the Root: Motherhood, Sexuality, and Male Dominance*. London: Pandora, 1989.

Flad, Mary M. "Tracing an Irish Widow's Journey: Immigration and Medical Care in the Mid-nineteenth Century." *Geoforum* 26, no. 3 (1995): 261–72.

Foucault, Michel. *Archaeology of Knowledge*. New York: Routledge, 1972.

———. *The Birth of a Clinic: An Archaeology of Medical Perception*. New York: Vintage, 1973.

———. *An Introduction*. Vol. 1 of *History of Sexuality*. New York: Vintage, 1978.

———. *Discipline and Punish: The Birth of the Prison*. New York: Vintage, 1979.

———. *Herculine Barbin: Being the Recently Discovered Memoirs of a Nineteenth-century French Hermaphrodite*. Brighton: Harvester Press, 1980.

———. *Power/Knowledge: Selected Interviews and Other Writings, 1972–1977*. New York: Pantheon, 1980.

———. "Questions on Geography." In *Power/Knowledge: Selected Interviews and Other Writings, 1972–1977*. New York: Pantheon, 1980.

———. "What Is Enlightenment?" In *The Foucault Reader*, ed. Paul Rabinow, 32–50. New York: Pantheon, 1984.

———. *The Care of the Self*. Vol. 3 of *The History of Sexuality*. New York: Vintage, 1988.

———. *The Use of Pleasure*. Vol. 2 of *The History of Sexuality*. New York: Vintage, 1990.

Frank, Arthur. *At the Will of the Body*. Boston: Houghton Mifflin, 1991.

———. *The Wounded Storyteller: Body, Illness, and Ethics*. Chicago: University of Chicago Press, 1995.

Frank, Gelya. "On Embodiment: A Case of Congenital Limb Deficiency in American Culture." In *Women with Disabilities: Essays in Psychology, Culture and Politics*, ed. Michelle Fine and Adrienne Asch. Philadelphia: Temple University Press, 1988.

Friedberg, Fred, and Leonard A. Jason. *Understanding Chronic Fatigue Syndrome:*

An Empirical Guide to Assessment and Treatment. Washington, D.C.: American Psychological Association, 2000.

Fuss, Diana. *Essentially Speaking.* New York: Routledge, 1989.

Gallaher, Carolyn. "Social Policy and the Construction of Need: A Critical Examination of the Geography of Needs Assessments for Low-income Women's Health." *Geoforum* 26, no. 3 (1995): 287–96.

Garber, Marjorie J. *Bisexuality and the Eroticism of Everyday Life.* New York: Routledge, 2000. (Originally published as *Vice Versa: Bisexuality and the Eroticism of Everyday Life.* New York: Simon and Schuster, 1995.)

Gatens, Moira. *Imaginary Bodies.* New York: Routledge, 1996.

Geertz, Clifford. *Local Knowledge.* New York: Basic, 1983.

Gibson-Graham, Julie-Kathy. *The End of Capitalism (as We Knew It): A Feminist Critique of Political Economy.* Oxford: Blackwell, 1996.

Glazer, Nona Y. "Servants to Capital: Unpaid Domestic Labor and Paid Work." *Review of Radical Political Economics* 16, no. 1 (1984): 61–87.

Gleeson, Brendan. *Geographies of Disability.* New York: Routledge, 1999.

Goffman, Erving. *Behaviour in Public.* London: Allen Lane, 1963.

———. *Stigma: Notes on the Management of Spoiled Identity.* Harmondsworth, U.K.: Penguin, 1968 [1963].

———. *Interaction Ritual: Essays on Face-to-Face Behavior.* Garden City, N.Y.: Doubleday, 1968.

Goldenberg, Naomi R. *Resurrecting the Body: Feminism, Religion, and Psychoanalysis.* New York: Crossroad, 1993.

Gordon, Colin. Afterword to *Power/Knowledge: Selected Interviews and Other Writings, 1972–1977.* New York: Pantheon, 1980.

Grosz, Elizabeth. "Inscriptions and Body-maps: Representations and the Corporeal." In *Feminine, Masculine and Representation,* ed. Terry Threadgold and Anne Cranny-Francis. Sydney, Aus.: Allen and Unwin, 1990.

———. "Body Images: Neurophysiology and Corporeal Mappings." In *Volatile Bodies: Toward a Corporeal Feminism.* Bloomington: Indiana University Press, 1994.

———. "The Body as Inscriptive Surface." In *Volatile Bodies: Toward a Corporeal Feminism.* Bloomington: Indiana University Press, 1994.

———. *Volatile Bodies: Toward a Corporeal Feminism.* Bloomington: Indiana University Press, 1994.

———. "Bodies and Knowledges: Feminism and the Crisis of Reason." In *Space, Time, and Perversion.* New York: Routledge, 1995.

———. "Bodies-Cities." In *Space, Time, and Perversion.* New York: Routledge, 1995.

———. *Space, Time, and Perversion.* New York: Routledge, 1995.

———. "Psychoanalysis and the Body." In *Feminist Theory and the Body: A Reader,* ed. Janet Price and Margrit Shildrick. New York: Routledge, 1998.

Grosz, Elizabeth, and Elspeth Probyn, eds. *Sexy Bodies: The Strange Carnalities of Feminism.* New York: Routledge, 1995.

Hall, Edward. " 'Blood, Brain and Bones': Taking the Body Seriously in the Geography of Health and Impairment." *Area* 32 (2000): 21–30.

Haraway, Donna. "Situated Knowledges: The Science Question in Feminism and the Privilege of Partial Perspective." *Feminist Studies* 14, no. 3 (1998): 575–99.

Hardie, Melissa Jane. " 'I Embrace the Difference': Elizabeth Taylor and the Closet." In *Sexy Bodies: The Strange Carnalities of Feminism*, ed. Elizabeth Grosz and Elspeth Probyn. New York: Routledge, 1995.

Harvey, David. "The Body as an Accumulation Strategy." *Environment & Planning D: Society & Space* 16 (1999): 401–21.

Hemmings, Clare. "Locating Bisexual Identities: Discourses of Bisexuality and Contemporary Feminist Theory." In *Mapping Desires*, ed. David Bell and Gill Valentine. New York: Routledge, 1995.

Henderson, Karla, and Barbara Ainsworth. "Researching Leisure and Physical Activity with Women of Color: Issues and Emerging Questions." *Leisure Sciences* 23, no. 1 (2001): 21–34.

Hennessy, Rosemary, and Chrys Ingraham, eds. *Materialist Feminism: A Reader in Class, Difference, and Women's Lives.* New York: Routledge, 1995.

Henriksson, Chris M. "Living with Continuous Muscular Pain—Patient Perspectives, Part 1: Encounters and Consequences." *Scandinavian Journal of Caring Science* 9 (1995): 67–76.

Herndl, Diane Price. *Invalid Women: Figuring Feminine Illness in American Fiction and Culture, 1840–1940.* Chapel Hill: University of North Carolina Press, 1993.

Hertz, Robert. *Death and the Right Hand.* New York: Cohen and West, 1960 [1909].

hooks, bell. "Choosing the Margin as a Space of Radical Openness." In *Yearning: Race, Gender, and Cultural Politics.* Boston: South End Press, 1990. Reprinted in *Women, Knowledge and Reality*, ed. Ann Garry and Marilyn Pearsall. New York: Routledge, 1996.

Howson, Alexandra. "Embodied Obligation: The Female Body and Health Surveillance." In *The Body in Everyday Life*, ed. Sarah Nettleton and Jonathan Watson. New York: Routledge, 1999.

Huyssen, Andreas. "Mapping the Postmodern." In *Feminism/Postmodernism*, ed. Linda J. Nicholson. New York: Routledge, 1990.

Imrie, Rob F. *Disability and the City: International Perspectives.* London: Paul Chapmen, 1996.

Isherwood, Lisa. *The Good News of the Body: Sexual Theology and Feminism.* Sheffield, U.K.: Sheffield University Press, 2000.

Jason, Leonard A., Judith A. Richman, Alfred W. Rademaker, Karen M. Jordon, Audrius V. Plioplys, Renee R. Taylor, William McCready, Cheng-Fang Huang, and Sigita Plioplys. "A Community-based Study of Chronic Fatigue Syndrome." *Archives of Internal Medicine (JAMA)* 159, no. 18 (October 11, 1999): http//archinte.ama-assn.org/issues/v159n18/full/ioi90161.html.

Jason, Leonard A., Renee R. Taylor, Zuzana Stepanek, and Sigita Plioplys. "Attitudes Regarding Chronic Fatigue Syndrome: The Importance of a Name." *Journal of Health Psychology* 6, no. 1 (2001): 61–71.

Johnson, Hillary. *Osler's Web: Inside the Labyrinth of the Chronic Fatigue Syndrome Epidemic.* New York: Crown, 1996.

Johnston, Lynda. "The Politics of the Pump: Hard Core Gyms and Women Body Builders." *New Zealand Geographer* 15, no. 3 (1995): 16–18.

————. "Flexing Femininity: Female Body Builders Refiguring 'The Body.' " *Gender, Place, and Culture* 3 (1996): 327–40.

Jones, Andrew. "(Re)producing Gender Relations." *Geoforum* 29 (1999): 451–74.

Jones, John Paul III, Heidi J. Nast, and Susan M. Roberts, eds. *Thresholds in Feminist Geography: Difference, Methodology, Representation*. Lanham, Md.: Rowman & Littlefield, 1997.

Jones, Kelvyn, and Graham Moon. "Medical Geography: Taking Space Seriously." *Progress in Human Geography*, 17 (1993): 515–24.

Jongbloed, Lyn. "Factors Influencing Employment Status of Women with Multiple Sclerosis." *Canadian Journal of Rehabilitation* 9 (1996): 213–22.

————. "Disability Income: The Experiences of Women with Multiple Sclerosis." *Canadian Journal of Occupational Therapy* 65 (1998): 193–201.

Katz, Cindi. "Playing the Field: Questions of Fieldwork in Geography." *Professional Geographer* 46 (1994): 67–72.

Kaufman, Sharon. "Illness, Biography, and the Interpretation of Self Following a Stroke." *Journal of Aging Studies* 2, no. 3 (1988): 217–27.

Keane, Angela, and Avril Horner. *Body Matters: Feminism, Textuality, Corporeality*. Manchester, U.K.: Manchester University Press, 2000.

Kearns, Robin A., and Alun E. Joseph. "Space in Its Place: Developing the Link in Medical Geography." *Social Science and Medicine* 37, no. 6 (1993): 711–17.

Keith, Michael, and Steve Pile, eds. *Place and the Politics of Identity*. New York: Routledge, 1993.

King, Debra Walker, ed. *Body Politics and the Fictional Double*. Bloomington: Indiana University Press, 2000.

Kirby, Sandra, and Kate McKenna. *Experience Research Social Change: Methods from the Margins*. Toronto: Garamond Press, 1989.

Kleinman, Arthur. *The Illness Narratives: Suffering, Healing, and the Human Condition*. New York: Basic, 1988.

Klimas, Nancy G., and Roberto Patarca, eds. *Disability and Chronic Fatigue Syndrome: Clinical, Legal, and Patient Perspectives*. New York: Haworth Press, 1997.

Kolb, Patricia. "Continuing to Care: Black and Latina Daughters' Assistance to Their Mothers in Nursing Homes." *Affilia* 15 (2000): 502–25.

Komaroff, Anthony L., and Laura R. Fagioli. "Medical Assessment of Fatigue and Chronic Fatigue Syndrome." In *Chronic Fatigue Syndrome: An Integrative Approach to Evaluation and Treatment*, ed. Mark A. Dematrack and Susan E. Abbey. New York: Guilford, 1996.

Komesaroff, Paul A., ed. *Troubled Bodies: Critical Perspectives on Postmodernism, Medical Ethics, and the Body*. Durham, N.C.: Duke University Press, 1995.

Kristeva, Julia. *Revolution in Poetic Language*. Trans. Margaret Walker. New York: Columbia University Press, 1984.

————. *Tales of Love*. Trans. Leon S. Roudiez. New York: Columbia University Press, 1987.

Krogh, Kari, and the Home Support Action Group, producers. "Beyond Four Walls." Report and video available through *http://www.ryerson.ca/kkrogh/report1/toc.html*.

Lawler, Jocalyn. *Behind the Screens: Nursing, Somology, and the Problem of the Body*. North American edition. Redwood City, Calif.: Benjamin/Cummings, 1993.

Lefebvre, Henri. *The Everyday Life of the Modern World.* Middlesex, U.K.: Penguin, 1968. English translation 1972.

———. *The Urban Revolution.* Paris: Gallimard, 1970.

Leslie, Deborah, and David Butz. " 'GM Suicide': Flexibility, Space, and the Injured Body." *Economic Geography* 74 (1998): 360–78.

Lesser, Ronnie C. "Objectivity as Masquerade." In *Disorienting Sexuality: Psychoanalytic Reappraisals of Sexual Identities,* ed. Thomas Domenici and Ronnie C. Lesser. New York: Routledge, 1995.

Levin, David Michael. "The Body Politic: The Embodiment of Praxis in Foucault and Habermas." *Praxis International* 9, no. 1–2 (July 1989): 112–32.

Lewis, Jane, and Barbara Meredith. *Daughters Who Care: Daughters Caring for Mothers at Home.* London: Routledge and Kegan Paul, 1988.

Litva, Andrea, and John Eyles. "Coming Out: Exposing Social Theory in Medical Geography." *Health & Place* 1 (1995): 5–14.

Litva, Andrea, Kay Peggs, and Graham Moon. "The Beauty of Health: Locating Young Women's Health and Appearance." In *Geographies of Women's Health,* ed. Isabel Dyck, Nancy Davis Lewis, and Sara McLafferty. New York: Routledge, 2001.

Lloyd, Genevieve. *The Man of Reason: 'Male' and 'Female' in Western Philosophy.* Minneapolis: University of Minnesota Press, 1984.

Longhurst, Robyn. *Bodies: Exploring Fluid Boundaries.* New York: Routledge, 2001.

Longhurst, Robyn, and Lynda Johnston. "Embodying Places and Emplacing Bodies: Pregnant Women and Women Body Builders." In *Feminist Thought in Aotearoa/ New Zealand,* ed. Rosemary DuPlessis and Lynne Alice. Auckland, N.Z.: Oxford University Press, 1998.

MacDonald, Eleanor. "The Trouble with Subjects: Feminism, Marxism, and the Questions of Poststructuralism." *Studies in Political Economy* 35 (1991): 43–71.

Malkki, Liisa. "Refugees and Exile: From 'Refugee Studies' to the National Order of Things." *Annual Review of Anthropology* 24 (1995): 495–524.

Marshall, Joan. "Borderlands and Feminist Ethnography." In *Feminist Geography in Practice: Research and Methods,* ed. Pamela Moss. London: Blackwell, 2002.

Martin, Cathy D. "More Than the Work: Race and Gender Differences in Caregiving Burden." *Journal of Family Issues* 21 (2000): 986–1005.

Martin, Emily. *The Woman in the Body: A Cultural Analysis of Reproduction.* 2nd ed. Boston: Beacon Press, 1992.

———. *Flexible Bodies: The Role of Immunity in American Culture from the Days of Polio to the Age of AIDS.* Boston: Beacon Press, 1994.

Massey, Doreen. *Spatial Divisions of Labour.* London: Macmillan, 1984.

———. "A Global Sense of Place." In *Space, Place, and Gender.* Minneapolis: University of Minnesota Press, 1995.

———. *Space, Place and Gender.* Minneapolis: University of Minnesota Press, 1995.

Mauss, Marcel. "Techniques of the Body." *Economy and Society* 2 (1973 [1934]): 70–88.

May, Robert. "Re-Reading Freud on Homosexuality." In *Disorienting Sexuality: Psychoanalytic Reappraisals of Sexual Identities,* ed. Thomas Domenici and Ronnie C. Lesser. New York: Routledge, 1995.

McDowell, Linda. "Towards an Understanding of the Gender Division of Urban Space." *Environment and Planning D; Society and Space* 1 (1983): 15–30.

————, ed. *Gender, Identity, and Space: Understanding Feminist Geographies.* Cambridge: Polity Press, 1999.

————. "In and Out of Place: Bodies and Embodiment." In *Gender, Identity, and Place: Understanding Feminist Geographies.* Oxford: Polity Press, 1999.

McDowell, Linda, and Gill Court. "Performing Work: Bodily Representations in Merchant Banks." *Environment and Planning D: Society and Space* 12 (1994): 727–50.

McLafferty, Sara, and Barbara Tempalski. "Restructuring and Women's Reproductive Health: Implications for Low Birthweight in New York City." *Geoforum* 26, no. 3 (1995): 309–23.

Merleau-Ponty, Maurice. *The Phenomenology of Perception.* New York: Routledge, 1999 [1962].

Miller, Baila. "Gender Differences in Spouse Management of the Caregiver Role." In *Circles of Care: Work and Identity in Women's Lives*, ed. Emily K. Abel and Margaret K. Nelson. New York: SUNY Press, 1990.

Miller, Nancy K. *Getting Personal: Feminist Occasions and Other Autobiographical Acts.* New York: Routledge, 1993.

Monaghan, Lee. "Creating 'The Perfect Body': A Variable Project." *Body & Society* 5, nos. 2 and 3 (1999): 267–90.

Money, John. *Gay, Straight, and In-Between: Sexology of Erotic Orientation.* New York: Oxford University Press, 1988.

Moraga, Cherríe, and Gloria Anzaldúa, eds. *This Bridge Called My Back: Writings by Radical Women of Color.* New York: Kitchen Table, Women of Color Press, 1986.

Moss, Pamela. "Negotiating Spaces in Home Environments: Older Women Living with Arthritis." *Social Science and Medicine* 45 (1997): 23–33.

————. "Autobiographical Notes on Chronic Illness." In *Mind and Body Spaces: Geographies of Disability, Illness, and Impairment*, ed. Ruth Butler and Hester Parr. New York: Routledge, 1999.

————. "Opening Up Discursive Space for Engaging Reflexive Methods." Presentation at the Annual Meeting of the Canadian Association of Geographers, St. Catharines, Ont., Canada (May 2000). Available from author, Faculty of Human and Social Development, University of Victoria, V8W 3P5.

————. " 'Not Quite Abled, Not Quite Disabled': Experiences of Being 'In Between' ME and the Academy." *Disability Studies Quarterly* 20 (2000): 287–93.

————. "Writing One's Life." In *Placing Autobiography in Geography*, ed. Pamela Moss. Syracuse, N.Y.: Syracuse University Press, 2001.

Moss, Pamela, and Isabel Dyck. "Inquiry into Environment and Body: Women, Work and Chronic Illness." *Environment & Planning D: Society & Space* 14 (1996): 737–53

————. "Body, Corporeal Space, and Legitimating Chronic Illness: Women Diagnosed with ME." *Antipode* 31 (1999): 372–97.

————. "Journeying through ME: Identity, the Body, and Women with Chronic Illness." In *Embodied Geographies: Spaces, Bodies, and Rites of Passage*, ed. Elizabeth Kenworthy Teather. New York: Routledge, 1999.

————. "Material Bodies Precariously Positioned: Working Women Diagnosed with Chronic Illness." In *Geographies of Women's Health*, ed. Isabel Dyck, Nancy Davis Lewis, and Sara McLafferty. New York: Routledge, 2001.

Moss, Pamela, and Margo Matwychuk. "Beyond Speaking as an 'As A' and Stating the 'Etc.': Toward a Praxis of Difference." *Frontiers* 21, no. 3 (2000): 82–104.

Moss, Pamela, and Martha McMahon. "Between a Flake and a Strident Bitch: Making 'It' Count in the Academy." *Resources for Feminist Research/Documentation sur la recherche féministe* 28, no. 1–2 (2000): 15–32.

Mouffe, Chantal. "Feminism, Citizenship, and Radical Democratic Politics." In *Feminists Theorize the Political*, ed. Judith Butler and Joan W. Scott. New York: Routledge, 1992.

————. "Post-Marxism: Democracy and Identity." *Environment & Planning D: Society and Space* 13 (1995): 259–65.

Munson, Peggy. "The Paradox of Lost Fingerprints: Metaphor and the Shaming of Chronic Fatigue Syndrome." In *Stricken: Voices from the Hidden Epidemic of Chronic Fatigue Syndrome*, ed. Peggy Munson. New York: Haworth Press, 2000.

Musafar, Fakir. "Body Play: State of Grace or Sickness?" In *Bodies under Siege: Self-Mutilation and Body Modification in Culture and Psychiatry*, ed. Armando R. Favvaza. Baltimore, Md.: Johns Hopkins University Press, 1996.

Nanda, Meera. " 'History Is What Hurts': A Materialist Feminist Perspective on the Green Revolution and Its Ecofeminist Critics." In *Materialist Feminism: A Reader in Class, Difference, and Women's Lives*, ed. Rosemary Hennessy and Chrys Ingraham. New York: Routledge, 1995.

Nast, Heidi. "Opening Remarks on 'Women in the Field.' " *Professional Geographer* 46 (1994): 54–66.

————. "The Body as 'Place': Reflexivity and Fieldwork in Kano, Nigeria." In *Places through the Body*, ed. Heidi J. Nast and Steve Pile. New York: Routledge, 1998.

Nast, Heidi J., and Steve Pile. "Introduction: MakingPlaceBodies." In *Places through the Body*, ed. Heidi J. Nast and Steve Pile. New York: Routledge, 1998.

————, eds. *Places through the Body*. New York: Routledge, 1998.

Natter, Wolfgang, and John Paul Jones III. "Identity, Space, and Other Uncertainties." In *Space and Social Theory: Interpreting Modernity and Postmodernity*, ed. Georges Benko and Ulf Strohmayer. Oxford: Blackwell, 1997.

Nelson, James B. *Body Theology*. Louisville: Westminster/John Knox Press, 1988.

Nettleton, Sarah, and Jonathan Watson, eds. *The Body in Everyday Life*. New York: Routledge, 1997.

Nicholson, Linda J., ed. *Feminism/Postmodernism*. New York: Routledge, 1990.

O'Brien, Mary. *The Politics of Reproduction*. Boston: Routledge and Kegan Paul, 1981.

O'Farrell, Mary Ann, and Lynne Vallone, eds. *Virtual Gender: Fantasies of Subjectivity and Embodiment*. Ann Arbor: University of Michigan Press, 1999.

Oliver, Mike. *Understanding Disability: From Theory to Practice*. Basingstoke, U.K.: Macmillan, 1996.

Paltial, Freda L. "The Disabled Women's Network in Canada." *Sexuality and Disability* 5, no. 1 (1997): 47–50.

Park, Deborah C., John P. Radford, and Michael H. Vickers. "Disability Studies in Human Geography." *Progress in Human Geography* 22 (1998): 208–33.

Parr, Hester. "Bodies and Psychiatric Medicine: Interpreting Different Geographies of Mental Health." In *Mind and Body Spaces: Geographies of Illness, Impairment, and Disability*, ed. Ruth Butler and Hester Parr. New York: Routledge, 1999.

Parr, Hester, and Chris Philo. "Mapping 'Mad' Identities." In *Mapping the Subject: Geographies of Cultural Transformation*, ed. Steve Pile and Nigel Thrift. New York: Routledge, 1995.

Pereira, Malin. *Embodying Beauty: Twentieth-century American Women Writers' Aesthetics*. New York: Garland, 2000.

Philo, Chris. "Staying In? Invited Comments on 'Coming Out': Exposing Social Theory in Medical Geography." *Health & Place* 2 (1996): 35–40.

Pile, Steve. "Human Agency and Human Geography Revisited: A Critique of 'New Models' of the Self." *Transactions of the Institute of British Geographers* 18 (1993): 122–39.

———. *The Body and the City: Psychoanalysis, Space, and Subjectivity*. New York: Routledge, 1996.

Pile, Steve, and Nigel Thrift. "Introduction." In *Mapping The Subject: Geographies of Cultural Transformation*, ed. Steve Pile and Nigel Thrift. New York: Routledge, 1995.

Pinder, Ruth. "Striking Balances: Living with Parkinson's Disease." In *Living with Chronic Illness: The Experiences of Patients and Their Families*, ed. Robert Anderson and Michael Bury. London: Hyman Unwin, 1988.

———. "Sick-but-fit or Fit-but-sick? Ambiguity and Identity in the Workplace." In *Exploring the Divide: Illness and Disability*, ed. Colin Barnes and Geoff Mercer. Leeds, U.K.: Disability Press, 1996.

Pratt, Geraldine. "Reflections on Poststructuralism and Feminist Empirics, Theory, and Practice." *Antipode* 25 (1993): 51–63.

Pratt, Geraldine, in collaboration with the Philippine Women Centre, Vancouver, Canada. "Inscribing Domestic Work on Filipina Bodies." In *Places through the Body*, ed. Heidi J. Nast and Steve Pile. New York: Routledge, 1998.

Price, Patricia L. "Bodies, Faith, and Inner Landscapes: Rethinking Change from the Very Local." *Latin American Perspectives* 26, no. 3 (1999): 37–59.

Pringle, Rosemary. *Secretaries Talk: Sexuality, Power, and Work*. London: Verso, 1989.

Probyn, Elspeth. "Travels in the Postmodern: Making Sense of the Local." In *Feminism/Postmodernism*, ed. Linda J. Nicholson. New York: Routledge, 1990.

———. *Sexing the Self: Gendered Positions in Cultural Studies*. New York: Routledge, 1993.

Ramazanoglu, Caroline. *Up against Foucault: Explorations of Some Tensions between Foucault and Feminism*. New York: Routledge, 1993.

Robinson, Ian. "Personal Narratives, Social Careers and Medical Courses: Analysing Life Trajectories in Autobiographies of People with Multiple Sclerosis." *Social Science and Medicine* 30 (1990): 1173–86.

Rodríguez Rust, Paula C. "Bisexuality: A Contemporary Paradox for Women." *Journal of Social Issues* 56, no. 2 (2000): 205–21.

Rose, Gillian. *Feminism and Geography: The Limits of Geographical Knowledge.* Minneapolis: University of Minnesota Press, 1993.

———. "Situating Knowledges: Positionality, Reflexivities and Other Tactics." *Progress in Human Geography* 21 (1997): 305–320.

Routledge, Paul. "The Third Space as Critical Engagement." *Antipode* 28 (1996): 399–419.

Russel, Kathryn. "A Value-Theoretic Approach to Childbirth and Reproductive Engineering." In *Materialist Feminism: A Reader in Class, Difference, and Women's Lives,* ed. Rosemary Hennessy and Chrys Ingraham. New York: Routledge, 1995.

Sawicki, Jana. *Disciplining Foucault: Feminism, Power, and the Body.* New York: Routledge, 1991.

Schoef, Brooke Grundfest. "Inscribing the Body Politic: Women and AIDS in Africa." In *Pragmatic Women and Body Politics,* ed. Margaret Lock and Patricia A. Kaufert. Cambridge: Cambridge University Press, 1998.

Scott, Joan W. "Experience." *Critical Inquiry* (summer 1991): 773–97.

———. "Experience." In *Feminists Theorize the Political,* ed. Judith Butler and Joan W. Scott. New York: Routledge, 1992.

Sharma, Ursula. "Bringing the Body Back into the (Social) Action: Techniques of the Body and the (Cultural) Imagination." *Social Anthropology* 4, no. 3 (1996): 251–63.

Sharp, Joanne P. "Gendering Nationhood: A Feminist Engagement with National Identity." In *Body/Space: Destabilizing Geographies of Gender and Sexuality,* ed. Nancy Duncan. New York: Routledge, 1996.

Shildrick, Margrit. *Leaky Bodies and Boundaries: Feminism, Postmodernism, and (Bio-) Ethics.* New York: Routledge, 1997.

Shildrick, Margrit, and Janet Price. "Breaking the Boundaries of the Broken Body." *Body and Society* 2, no. 4 (1996): 93–113.

Shilling, Chris. *The Body and Social Theory.* Thousand Oaks, Calif.: Sage, 1993.

Showalter, Elaine. *Hystories: Hysterical Epidemics and Modern Media.* New York: Columbia University Press, 1997.

Singleton, Judy. "Women Caring for Elderly Family Members: Shaping Non-traditional Work and Family Initiatives." *Journal of Comparative Family Studies* 31 (2000): 367–75.

Slack, Sandy. "I Am More Than My Wheels." In *Disability and Discourse,* ed. Mairian Corker and Sally French. London: Open University Press, 1999.

Soja, Edward W. "The Socio-Spatial Dialectic." *Annals of the Association of American Geographers* 70 (1980): 207–25.

———. "The Trialectics of Spatiality." In *Thirdspace: Journeys to Los Angeles and Other Real-and-Imagined Places.* London: Blackwell, 1996.

———. *Thirdspace: Journeys to Los Angeles and Other Real-and-Imagined Places.* Oxford: Blackwell, 1996.

Spivak, Gayatri Chakravorty. "Can the Subaltern Speak?" In *Colonial Discourses and Post-Colonial Theory: A Reader,* ed. Patrick Williams and Laura Chrisman. Hertfordshire, U.K.: Harvester Wheatsheaf, 1994.

Stone, Sharon Dale. "The Myth of Bodily Perfection." *Disability and Society,* 10 (1995): 413–24.

Storper, Michael, and Richard Walker. *The Capitalist Imperative*. Oxford: Blackwell, 1989.

Storr, Merl, ed. *Bisexuality: A Critical Reader*. New York: Routledge, 2000.

Strong, Jenny, Roderick Ashton, David Chant, and Tess Cramond. "An Investigation of the Dimensions of Chronic Low Back Pain: The Patients' Perspectives." *British Journal of Occupational Therapy* 57 (1994): 204–8.

Swift, Karen J., and Michael Birmingham. "Location, Location, Location: Restructuring and the Everyday Lives of 'Welfare Moms.' " In *Restructuring Caring Labour: Discourse, State Practice, and Everyday Life*, ed. Sheila M. Neysmith. Toronto: Oxford University Press, 2000.

Teather, Elizabeth Kenworthy, ed. *Embodied Geographies: Spaces, Bodies, and Rites of Passage*. New York: Routledge, 1999.

Terry, Jennifer. "Anxious Slippages between 'Us' and 'Them': A Brief History of the Scientific Search for Homosexual Bodies." In *Deviant Bodies*, ed. Jennifer Terry and Jacqueline Urla. Bloomington: Indiana University Press, 1995.

Tong, Rosemarie. *Feminist Approaches to Bioethics: Theoretical Reflections and Practical Applications*. Boulder, Colo.: Westview Press, 1997.

Turner, Bryan S. *The Body and Society*. 2nd ed. Oxford: Basil Blackwell, 1996.

Underhill-Sem, Yvonne. " 'The Baby Is Turning': Child-bearing in Wanigela, Oro Province, Papua New Guinea." In *Geographies of Women's Health*, ed. Isabel Dyck, Nancy Davis Lewis, and Sara McLafferty. New York: Routledge, 2001.

Valentine, Gill. "People Like Us: Negotiating Sameness and Difference in the Research Process." In *Feminist Geography in Practice: Research and Methods*, ed. Pamela Moss, 116–26. London: Blackwell, 2002.

Vash, Carolyn. "Employment Issues for Women with Disabilities." *Rehabilitation Literature* 43, nos. 7–8 (1982): 198–207.

Verillo, Erica F., and Lauren M. Gellman. *Chronic Fatigue Syndrome: A Treatment Guide*. New York: Quality Medical Publishing, 1998.

Vogel, Lise. *Marxism and the Oppression of Women: Toward a Unitary Theory*. New Brunswick, N.J.: Rutgers University Press, 1983.

Walby, Sylvia. *Gender Transformations*. New York: Routledge, 1996.

Warin, Megan, Frances Baum, Elizabeth Kalucy, Charlie Murray, and Bronwyn Veale. "The Power of Place: Space and Time in Women's and Community Health Centres in South Australia." *Social Science and Medicine* 50 (2000): 1863–75.

Weiss, Gail. *Body Images: Embodiment as Intercorporeality*. New York: Routledge, 1999.

Wendell, Susan. *The Rejected Body: Feminist Philosophical Reflections on Disability*. New York: Routledge, 1996.

Williams, Simon J., and Gillian A. Bendelow. "Bodily Control: Body Techniques, Intercorporeality and the Embodiment of Social Action." In *The Lived Body: Sociological Themes, Embodied Issues*. New York: Routledge, 1998.

———. "Pain and the Dys-Appearing Body." In *The Lived Body: Sociological Themes, Embodied Issues*. New York: Routledge, 1998.

———. "Sociology and the 'Problem' of the Body." In *The Lived Body: Sociological Themes, Embodied Issues*. New York: Routledge, 1998.

———. *The Lived Body: Sociological Themes, Embodied Issues.* New York: Routledge, 1998.

Wilson, David, and Pamela Moss. "Spatiality Studies in Urban Geography." In *Research in Urban Sociology,* vol. 4, ed. Ray Hutchinson. Greenwich, Conn.: JAI Press, 1997.

Wilson, Elizabeth. "Is Transgression Transgressive?" In *Activating Theory: Lesbian, Gay, Bisexual Politics,* ed. Joseph Bristow and Angelia R. Wilson. London: Lawrence and Wishart, 1993.

Wise, Sue. "Sexing Elvis." *Women's Studies International Forum* 7, no. 1 (1984): 13–17.

Witz, Anne. "Whose Body Matters? Feminist Sociology and the Corporeal Turn in Sociology and Feminism." *Body and Society* 6, no. 2 (2000): 1–24.

"Women in the Field." *Professional Geographer* 46 (1995): 54–102.

Yeatman, Anna. "A Feminist Theory of Social Differentiation." In *Feminism/Postmodernism,* ed. Linda J. Nicholson. New York: Routledge, 1990.

Yelin, Edward H. "Gender, Disability, and Employment." *Occupational Medicine* 8 (1993): 849–58.

Young, Iris Marion. "The Ideal of Community and the Politics of Difference." In *Feminism/Postmodernism,* ed. Linda J. Nicholson. New York: Routledge, 1990.

———. "The Scaling of Bodies and the Politics of Identity." In *Justice and the Politics of Difference.* Princeton, N.J.: Princeton University Press, 1990.

———. *Throwing Like a Girl and Other Essays.* Bloomington: Indiana University Press, 1990.

Yuval-Davis, Nira. *Gender and Nation.* London: Sage, 1997.

Index

Abbey, Susan, 39
accommodation, 116, 119
agency, 21, 48
agoraphobia, 100, 151
alternative medicine, 6–7
analysis: coding, 80; mappings of interviews, 80; of transcriptions, 81;
  seduction in, 62–65; and social location, 78; and truth, 63
Anderson, Vivienne, 40
anorexia nervosa, 43, 61–62, 97
antitheory, 58–59
arthritis, 93, 96, 139
autobiography, 20; writing, 59–60, 77
autonomy, 196n9

Bendelow, Gillian, 21, 24–25, 26
Benhabib, Seyla, 61
binary. *See* dualism(s)
bodies: disabled, 59–60; discursive and
  material, 37, 40, 113; entities, 26,
  36–44; ill, 36–44; representational
  and material, 12; and space, 56
"bodies in context," 51, 66, 125–26,
  132, 133, 155, 166, 168; definition
  of, 52; and identity, 138, 140; and
  self, 142; and spatiality, 66; as specific, 59; as tension, 56
bodily activities, 43, 61–62, 133, 168
bodily control, 24, 111, 153
bodily limits, 60, 113, 116, 122–23,
  132, 134; and environment, 153,
  156, 158–59; and self, 136
bodily sensation, 35–36, 41, 105
body: alterity, 61; and anorexia nervosa,

43; biological aspects of, 20; chaotic,
112–13, 118; concrete, 41, 48–49;
concrete and specific, 27–28; constitutive with space, 47; cultural, 41,
43; destabilized/destabilizing, 93,
115, 118, 158; destabilized material,
42, 96, 98; deviant, 38, 93; disabled,
108; disabling aspects of the material,
108; discursive, 14, 31; discursive
and material in context, 56–57; discussion of body made *specific*, 56–57;
docile, 63; ideal, 22; ideal(ized), 62,
96; and identity, 26, 36, 37; invalid,
39, 85, 107, 120; made *specific*, 54,
99; material aspects of, 21; metaphor
of, 110–11; modification, 41–42;
non-specific, 36; ontological differences in ill, 101–2; "perfect," 177n3;
pre-discursive, 61, 88; pre-mattered,
191n26; process of being made *specific*, 158–62; regulated, 63; sculpted, 42; sensorial, 36–37; sensual, 60,
67; as site of oppression, 126; as site
of resistance, 126; and space, 46–47;
specific, 29, 33, 34, 37, 41, 44, 46,
48, 51, 55, 57, 61, 67, 85, 93, 102,
138, 158, 159, 161, 163, 166; in
transition, 22; unified account of, 64.
See also theories of the body
body-based materiality, 60
body image, 133, 177n5
body play, 41
Bondi, Liz, 48
borders: embodying of, 128; flexibility,
  115; fluidity of, 107–8, 122–23,

About the Authors

Pamela Moss is a feminist geographer in the Faculty of Human and Social Development at the University of Victoria, Canada. She teaches in the Studies in Policy & Practice Program, an interdisciplinary graduate program for professionals in health and social services. Her research interests include body politics, feminist theory, autobiography, and women's experiences of chronic illness. She is also a community activist involved with creating innovative housing programs for women in crisis.

Isabel Dyck is a social geographer in the School of Rehabilitation Sciences and faculty associate, Women's Studies, the University of British Columbia, Canada. She teaches qualitative methodology, geographies of disability, and feminist theories of the body. Her research interests include women with chronic illness, and immigrant women and girls' resettlement narratives related to family reconstitution, school and youth identity, and health care access and experiences.